HEALTH RACE & ETHNICITY

Edited by
Thomas Rathwell
David Phillips

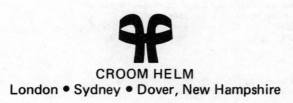

CROOM HELM
London • Sydney • Dover, New Hampshire

©1986 Tom Rathwell and David Phillips
Croom Helm Ltd, Provident House, Burrell Row,
Beckenham, Kent BR3 1AT
Croom Helm Australia Pty Ltd, Suite 4, 6th Floor,
64-76 Kippax Street, Surry Hills, NSW 2010, Australia

British Library Cataloguing in Publication Data

Health, race and ethnicity.
   1. Minorities – Medical care 2. Race
   discrimination
   I. Rathwell, Tom II. Phillips, David
   362.1'089   RA418

   ISBN 0-7099-4221-4

Croom Helm, 51 Washington Street, Dover,
New Hampshire 03820, USA

Library of Congress Cataloging in Publication Data
Main entry under title:

Health, race and ethnicity.
   Based on a conference on ethnic health issues, held
at the University of Leeds' Nuffield Centre for Health
Services Studies in July 1983, organized by the
Institute of British Geographers' Medical Geography
study group.

   Includes index.
   1. Minorities–medical care–congresses.
2. Discrimination in medical care–congresses.
3. Social medicine–congresses. I. Rathwell, Tom,
1944–   . II. Phillips, David, 1953–   .
III. Conference on ethnic health issues (1983:
University of Leeds' Nuffield Centre for Health
Services Studies) IV. Institute of British Geographers.
Medical Geography study group. (DNLM: 1. Delivery of
health care–congresses. 2. Ethnic groups–congresses.
3. Health–congresses. WA 300 H434 1983)
RA563.M56H43   1986   362.1'089   85-28027
ISBN 0-7099-4221-4

Printed and bound in Great Britain
by Billing & Sons Limited, Worcester.

CONTENTS

List of Contributors
Preface
Acknowledgements

1.   ETHNICITY AND HEALTH: INTRODUCTION AND
     DEFINITIONS
     David Phillips and Tom Rathwell   1

PART ONE: HEALTH, RACE AND CULTURE: THEMES
AND ISSUES

2.   RACE, DISEASE AND HEALTH
     Richard Cooper   21

3.   ETHNIC DIFFERENCE IN DISEASE -
     AN EPIDEMIOLOGICAL PERSPECTIVE
     Ranjit Bandaranayake   80

4.   THE POLITICS OF ETHNIC MINORITY HEALTH
     STUDIES
     Maggie Pearson   100

PART TWO: HEALTH CARE FOR ETHNIC MINORITIES
NEEDS AND PROVISION

5.   BLACK PEOPLE'S HEALTH: A DIFFERENT
     APPROACH?
     Jenny Donovan   117

6.   ETHNIC STATUS AND MENTAL ILLNESS IN
     URBAN AREAS
     John Giggs   137

Contents

7.   HEALTH CARE AND ETHNIC MINORITIES IN
     DENMARK
     Marianne Lauridsen   175

8.   INNER CITY RESIDENTS, ETHNIC MINORITIES
     AND PRIMARY HEALTH CARE IN THE WEST MIDLANDS
     Mark Johnson   192

9.   DOES RACE AFFECT HOSPITAL USE?
     John Griffith, Peter Wilson and Philip
     Tedeschi   213

10. NUTRITIONAL STATUS OF BLACK COMMUNITIES IN
     THE EASTERN CAPE - SOUTH AFRICA, ASSESSMENT
     AND POLICY RECOMMENDATIONS
     Rob Fincham   236

11. ETHNICITY AND HEALTH: AN AGENDA FOR
     PROGRESSIVE ACTION!
     Tom Rathwell and David Phillips   255

Index   271
                                              279

LIST OF CONTRIBUTORS

DR RANJIT BANDARANAYKE a is Specialist in Community Medicine (Environmental Health), Bradford Health Authority, and Lecturer in the Department of Community Medicine and General Practice, University of Leeds, Leeds, England.

DR RICHARD COOPER is a physician at Cook County Hospital, Chicago, United States of America, and an active member of the International Committee Against Racism.

MS JENNY DONOVAN is a Researcher in the Department of Geography and Earth Science, Queen Mary College, London, England.

MR ROB FINCHAM is a Lecturer in the Department of Geography, Rhodes University, Grahamstown, South Africa.

DR JOHN GRIFFITH is Pattullo Collegiate Professor in Hospital Administration, School of Public Health, University of Michigan, Ann Arbor, Michigan, United States.

DR JOHN GIGGS is a Senior Lecturer in the Department of Geography, University of Nottingham, Nottingham, England.

DR MARK JOHNSON is a Senior Research Fellow in the Centre for Research in Ethnic Relations, University of Warwick, Coventry, England.

MS MARIANNE LAURIDSEN is a civil servant in the Ministry of the Interior, Government of Denmark, Copenhagen, Denmark, and is now currently on secondment as Chief of Division (Planning), Statens Seruminstitut.

List of Contributors

MS MAGGIE PEARSON is Lecturer in Medical Sociology, Department of General Practice, University of Liverpool, and lately Director of the Centre of Ethnic Minority Health Studies, Bradford, England.

DR DAVID PHILLIPS is a Lecturer in the Department of Geography, University of Exeter, Exeter, England.

MR TOM RATHWELL is a Lecturer in the Nuffield Centre for Health Services Studies, Department of Social Policy and Health Services Studies, University of Leeds, Leeds, England.

DR PHILIP TEDESCHI is an Assistant Professor in the Department of Hospital Administration, School of Public Health, University of Michigan, Ann Arbor, Michigan, United States.

DR PETER WILSON is Vice President of the Michigan Hospital Association, Michigan, United States.

PREFACE

This book results from papers presented to a
Conference on Ethnic Health Issues, held at the
University of Leeds' Nuffield Centre for Health
Services Studies in July 1983. After the
conference authors revised and up-dated their
contributions and the two editors, who assisted in
the Conference, undertook to compile this book.
The conference itself was organised by the Institute
of British Geographers' Medical Geography Study
Group and the participants included, in addition to
geographers, a wide range of professionals with an
interest in health and health care: doctors,
epidemiologists, administrators and academics from
many other cognate disciplines. Therefore,
although a number of the contributions in this book
have a geographical theme this is generally but one
dimension in a subject as wide and cross-
disciplinary as it is multicultural. The
interdisciplinary nature of much of the work is of
great importance: we regard the contents as of
interest to physicians, health services planners,
nurses (especially community nurses),
physiotherapists, health services managers, social
biologists and many other professionals. We discuss
some of the interdisciplinary linkages in chapter
one.
      The development and nature of geographical and
other interest in the subject matter is discussed
below but it is important to point out now that
medical geographers have for sometime now been
interested in matters of social relevance related to
health and health care. This interest is of
especial concern, of course, when associated with
the distribution of health and health related
phenomena and access (social or spatial) to
facilities. However, before considering this in
more specific terms, we feel as editors that there
are a number of important issues to be introduced in
relation to the use of accepted or acceptable

definitions in the subject area of ethnicity and health. We are aware that this can become contentious and that to an extent terms are used (sometimes incorrectly) interchangeably and the terminology differs to an extent in different countries. We have tried to discuss this definitional issue as objectively as possible in the introductory chapter, but we do appreciate that our observations are necessarily influenced by our perceptions and, therefore, others may well wish to challenge us on these grounds. In the end, however, it is the reader who must decide on the validity or otherwise of our case.

ACKNOWLEDGEMENTS

We are grateful, as editors, to our fellow contributors for their patience, co-operation and effort in this project. Also a special thanks to Margaret Rathwell, who diligently read through the penultimate version of the manuscript. Without this help the book would contain far more errors than it does; for those that remain we accept full responsibility.

Finally, we are especially indebted to Sarah Barklam at the Nuffield Centre for Health Services Studies, University of Leeds for the secretarial skills required to transform this collection of papers into the completed manuscript for publication.

TOM RATHWELL
DAVID PHILLIPS

Chapter 1

ETHNICITY AND HEALTH: INTRODUCTION AND DEFINITIONS

David Phillips and Tom Rathwell

BACKGROUND

The first major perplexity concerns the use of terms
such as race and ethnicity. 'Race', in a dictionary
definition, suggests groups of people having or
supposed to have common ancestors. It exists as a
sociological construct but some authors have also
assumed or attempted to prove that it has a
biological or genetic component. The debate about
this fact of 'race' has become contentious and, as
Richard Cooper ably summarises in the following
chapter, the idea that race in a genetic or
biological sense determines health is now
discredited for all but a very small minority of
specific ailments. In general and lay terms, race
has come to be synonymous with skin colour. In
biological or genetic terms with regard to health,
this is obviously not particularly helpful since
there are as many physiological and health
variations occurring amongst persons with the same
skin colouring as between colours. Nevertheless, a
particularly invidious period of academic and
political history was associated with a belief in
racial determinism and particularly as regards
superiority or inferiority of races in physique,
intelligence and potential. This unfortunate trait
was particularly evident in some writing of the
nineteenth and early twentieth centuries and linked
to an extent with the history of colonialism.
Gobineau [1] provides an illustration of the types
of arguments portrayed in those days to justify such
beliefs and Zubaida [2] explains why it is necessary
to be aware of such an historical context which
perhaps underlies much of todays misunderstanding.
Cooper's chapter also illustrates this point.
      Race as a biological or genetic tool of
analysis has now, as stated, been largely
discredited and only a handful of unusual and

specific diseases seem to have racial correlations [3]. It is now generally accepted in the scientific community as proven that all humans are genetically similar except in terms of susceptibility to a few rare diseases some of which Cooper discusses. However, race does have validity as a social construct as it is strongly related to life chances and opportunities in many countries in the world. Stone puts this succinctly "the classical sociologists understood the fundamental point: the study of race and ethnic relations has little to do with biological 'race' and a lot to do with patterns of social relationships and structures of power and domination" [4].

Nevertheless, it seems that "theories of culture based on biological or racial determinism have a superficial and dangerous plausibility, so it is important to recognise that they are based on pseudo-science" [5]. In the early nineteenth century struggle against the slave trade, abolitionists came up against assertions of assured superiority of one race over another by Thomas Carlyle, and racial determinism also to an extent infected some abolitionists themselves: they were helping those who could not protect themselves. Bujra points out that it should be evident today that the infinite variety and changeability of cultural forms must remove facile generalisations based on fixed biological types. Some of the classical sociologist-anthropologists referred to above, and others such as Durkheim writing at the end of the nineteenth century, were eventually able to argue that social and cultural phenomena cannot be explained in simple reductionist terms but must be explained in their own terms. Therefore a social phenomenon (such as ethnic differences in health or health care) manifestly requires a sociological or societal explanation [6]. However it may remain difficult to convince some policy makers that this is the case although, fortunately, there exist sufficient enlightened professionals to ensure that the process of developing this belief will continue.

Jenny Donovan, in addition to her chapter in this book, has provided a useful discussion about the confusing use of terminology in this sphere of research [7]. As editors we recognise that, to an extent, the definitions of terms and substitutions of one word for another is often a matter of semantic nuances, but her contribution is helpfully clear. She suggests that 'minority', 'ethnic' or

'ethnic minority' may be used to describe any group
of people who share a cultural heritage but are not
part of the majority, and who may experience varying
degrees of discrimination.
     This helps to move terminology on from race-
racism to recognise the influence of shared culture,
social   factors   and   the   like.   Nevertheless, the
flow of information from academic publication to the
lay publications helped sustain 'race' rather than
ethnicity   as   the   unity   of debate.   Husband's
observation of this is important since the former
term has a sort of scientific permanency
"characterised   by   genetic   determination and
transmission, rather than plasticity inherent in
ethnicity with its basis in culture" [8]. It is
therefore important to be aware of the shortcomings
mentioned earlier which appertain to some aspects of
sociology and particularly the pseudo-science in
this area of research.
     The terms 'black', 'black people' and black
culture are   today   more generally acceptable in
Britain and North America than often inaccurate
terms such as 'coloured', 'negro' or 'Indian'.
Colour is an obvious distinguishing characteristic
of many minority groups in Europe and North America,
including Turkish, Cyprist, Vietnamese, Filipino,
Hispanic and other people, to name but a few.
However, colour does not necessarily readily
distinguish groups such as Irish, Welsh, Bretons,
Basques, Jews or gypsies all of whom may validly be
considered as ethnic minorities in some cases and
who may face problems with regard to health and
health care in some circumstances similar to those
of other minorities although, on the whole, their
problems will tend to be very much fewer than those
of groups distinguishable because of colour. This
reminds us that the question of ethnicity is, all
the same, a multi-faceted issue. Ahmed provides a
very useful overview of the inherent, perhaps even
unconscious racism of many words and phrases, and
indicates that the academic and 'popular' use of
terms may often be at odds [9].
     Within this book, the scale of numbers of
people affected by various forms of discrimination
and disadvantage vary. Lauridsen, for example,
talks of Denmark where ethnic minorities are
relatively small; Fincham at the other extreme is
dealing with the health circumstances of a majority
group, the black population of the Eastern Cape in
South Africa. Here, a racially distinct white
minority have important social, economic and

3

political advantages whilst the black majority are subjugated in these terms. The nature of the problems faced by these people will often differ considerably in scale and cause (if not so much in effect) from those faced by ethnic minority groups of, say, African, Caribbean or Asian descent in Britain or America.

Quite often, and particularly in Britain, the term 'immigrant' is used to describe members of ethnic minorities [10]. It is interesting to consider that, historically, this term was often applied to white immigrants to the United States whereas, today, the term will generally be found more commonly in Europe where more recent labour migration has occurred and where it refers on the whole to black immigration. However, when the term immigrant 'hangs over' to describe people who have not been born outside the country, its use is not logical. As Donovan points out, the use of the word is increasingly inappropriate in Britain, for example, as the majority of non-whites have been born there. Even in its 'census' meaning, the term refers to a highly diverse population by no means all of whom are of so-called 'New Commonwealth' (and, by implication, black) origin. The persistence of the term can have perjorative overtures suggesting alien or outsider; it also has implications that immigration may not be a one-way process and that non-assimilation or non-integration (and eventual return migration) may be desired. Marianne Lauridsen aptly discusses this matter in her chapter with regard to the situation in Denmark.

That differentials among ethnic groups exist because of social and economic differences should, perhaps, become even more evident in health and health care than in any other sphere of human relations. Manifest differences in health amongst ethnic groups, because not genetically determined, must be influenced by the social, economic and physical environments in which individuals and families live. Therefore, poor health and health care may be associatied with a range of other indices of disadvantage: low income, poor housing, low education and inadequate nutrition. If disadvantaged at home or at work as ethnic minorities often seem to be [11], then the familiar circle-of-poverty may well operate. However, it is important to remember that such cyclical deprivation does not necessarily relate to a culture of poverty accepted by minorities but rather to a position of economic and social disadvantage in terms of the political economy of many nations. Health care, for example, is often provided by the state which may be insensitive to, or overtly unaware of, specific needs of minorities or which may be unwilling or unable to distribute resources fairly within the existing political and economic framework. This higher level of analysis can be related at a practical level to questions of social and allocative justice referred to later.

With regard to this book, the editors and individual authors are aware that a particularly important and sensitive issue is being discussed by a group consisting mainly of white researchers investigating the health and welfare of black or other non-white ethnic groups. Maggie Pearson's chapter is particularly clear in explaining the potential shortcomings inherent in such a situation, pointing out the intrinsic dangers of developing white research into black people's health which may, in its avowed detachment and adherence to 'scientific objectivity', avoid indicting society which is guilty of racism, the fundamental root of the situation. As Pearson points out, the divorce of research from positive or committed action is understandably viewed with increasing suspicion and hostility on the part of black people who are usually the subject of increasing amounts of research, but rarely are consulted or involved in undertaking such research. In the concluding chapter we try to indicate some specific policy measures which may be applied and it is to be ardently hoped that these do not become yet another addition to the academic 'paper mountain'.

The question may be posed as to whether the value or validity of the research is reduced by the nature of the researcher. It is doubtful whether this can be resolved to the satisfaction of all parties but it does seem that the relative lack of black people researching into this topic represents a form of intellectual apartheid and, in western Europe at any rate, is yet another indicator of disadvantage. The educational system (arguably reflecting society's values) has allowed or encouraged relatively fewer people from ethnic groups to become 'academically qualified' in this field of research. It is, of course, ironic to consider the case of the British National Health Service (NHS) which has for a long time been strongly supported by doctors trained abroad and by nurses and ancillary staff belonging to ethnic minorities. It is argued by some that the fact

5

that most of these individuals are at the lower paid
end of the NHS is symbolic of continued disadvantage
and exploitation. This lower end of the health
service includes the medically qualified staff who
may not progress up the career hierarchy or who may
be forced to work in the less popular specialties.

Donovan also notes that there has been
relatively little contribution from the black
populations of Britain to the published research in
health care in the professional press [12] which is
in spite of the number of workers in the health
service from these groups. Consequently, it is
possible to argue that research has in part been
biased, concentrating on the unusual diseases or
illnesses which interest white doctors and
governments, such as rickets, tuberculosis and
sickle-cell anaemia. Ailments and problems
afflicting the majority of people in ethnic groups
have been ignored, particularly the pervasive nature
of disadvantage and discrimination in health care
(deliberate or accidental), and the links with the
large and growing literature on race relations.
Indeed, the concentrations on unusual illnesses or
on specific relatively rare diseases may, in fact,
have the effect of singling out some groups of
people as 'problems' [13]. McNaught also notes with
some surprise the lack of concern and knowledge in
the NHS about the interaction between health
services, race relations and status [14]. To this
extent, some of the papers in this book are very
timely and we return in the final chapter to the
issues of how to develop policy intitiatives and
provide a catalogue for positive action to redress
this imbalance.

It is pertinent, perhaps, to point out that in
Britain and in some other countries, until recently,
much research on attitudes and problems of ethnic
minorities has tended to omit wholly or partly
health and health care or to concentrate on unusual
aspects suggested above [15-18]. Recently, however,
British publications have generally become more
aware of this deficiency and have focused on a
number of aspects of health care and ethnicity,
sometimes concentrating on specific problems but
also dealing with aspects which involve larger
numbers of . sufferers such as mental
disorders [19,20] and in addition covering wider
matters such as the provision of services. Many of
these themes are illustrated in Johnson's
bibliography [21]. Elsewhere, and particularly in

the United States there has grown over a longer period a literature on health and ethnicity as Cooper's paper and other references illustrate [22,23].

SOME CROSS-DISCIPLINARY INTERESTS

This book originated from a conference arranged principally by medical geographers but many of the contributors came from other disciplines and professions. The growth of a 'geographical' focus on this subject is discussed below but here it may be of interest to highlight some of the considerable cross-disciplinary and cross-professional interest which has grown in ethnic health issues.

The concern of many medical practitioners and researchers has already been mentioned but in some ways this has perhaps been one of the most restrictive involvements. The tendency of many doctors has been to seek medical solutions to what are regarded as medical problems, therefore emphasising the 'medical model' of care. This model often has only limited relevance in the exploration and amelioration of socially and personally-based phenomena. Therefore, the image and expectations of what medical involvement and intervention could and should aim for are changing. Perhaps the profession for whom this changing role of 'medical' participation has the greatest implications is the group of paramedical and allied workers at the primary care level. The trend in many societies towards community care (usually linked with the deinstitutionalisation of much previously hospital-based treatment and care) has made it essential that community-level workers are alerted to social and political as well as medical aspects of their jobs. They are no longer seen to have the sole right to active intervention in 'problems'. Community nurses, public health nurses, occupational therapists, chiropodists and many other allied workers today are increasingly likely to meet ethnic minorities in their own homes to view first hand their situations and to be able to identify developments and potential breakdowns in care and communications.

These workers have become particularly important in introducing a range of official and other services to members of ethnic groups. Therefore, that awareness of the wider social and economic contexts in which they are working is

essential.   This is particularly so for the care of
groups   who   are   especially   vulnerable   in any
societies, such as the elderly, and the mentally ill
or   mentally   handicapped.   Being   a   member of an
ethnic   minority   almost   certainly   compounds such
elements   of   disadvantage and community workers are
increasingly   aware   of   this.   There is evidence to
suggest,   for   example,   that   the elderly of ethnic
groups   in Britain are disadvantaged in their access
to   health   care   whilst there is little information
relating   to   'levels   of   professional knowledge of
their needs' [24].   There is ample reason to suppose
that   the   situation   is   similar in other countries
covered in this book.
        With regard to the compounding of disadvantage,
it   is important to be aware that the ethnic elderly
can   receive   the   most   ineffective   responses from
society,   as   they   are   further   disadvantaged in a
group which is already in a relatively weak position
in   society.   Social   gerontologists   have   for long
recognised the vulnerable nature of the elderly, but
only   recently   is   the   special position of elderly
members   of ethnic groups becoming evident.   McNeely
and   Cohen's   edited   volume   provides   useful
consideration of ageing in   minority   groups [25].
They   point   out   race   and   ethnicity   as   critical
factors   in   low   take-up   of many services and they
identify   language   and other barriers to care.   The
resistence   to   acknowledging   race   as   a   relevant
variable   on   the   part   of   those   charged with the
design   and   implementation   of   programmes can be a
major shortcoming.   Overall, they stress the need to
create   culturally - responsive programmes sensitive
to   the   needs of diverse groups.   This can probably
only   be   achieved   by   active interdisciplinary co-
operation.
        Such   a recognition gains even   more   importance
today than   in the past with the growing reliance on
'community care'.   Members of ethnic groups as much
as   anyone else will tend to favour the provision of
care   in   its   broadest sense (which includes a wide
range   of   services)   in   familiar   moral and social
settings in the community [26].   This is perhaps the
key   to successful future social work amongst ethnic
minorities   who   are often members of what some have
more   generally   called   'undervalued'   groups of
clients.   A feature of provision for such people is
that   professionals   must   try   to   understand the
situations   in   which   these   individuals find
themselves rather   than trying to take charge. They
must   attempt to focus on the individual rather than

on some official master plan [27]. However, it may be very difficult for some professionals, trained in the active interventionist mode, to be able to adopt such a stance but it is well worth striving for. It may become increasingly difficult to achieve as it requires time and patience, commodities in short supply when restrictions on public expenditure in many countries mean that the time spent with any client or family has to be rationed. In additon, 'successful casework' for some professionals may be measured in terms which do not really reflect success from the point of view of the client (that is, the clearing of caseloads rather than adequate solving of problems).

It is hoped that this book will be of interest to professional medical administration and community physicians who are in positions to influence locally the allocation of resources and the establishment of 'objectives' for services. Perhaps some of the intentional or unintentional racism in the British NHS (as an example) will be tempered by increasing the input at a planning stage of consultation from consumers who are affected by local services [28]. It is professions at this level who need to be aware of ethnic issues and this theme is returned to in the concluding chapter.

Academics, too, other than medical geographers, medical sociologists, health economists and the like have diverse and longstanding interest in the subject matter of the book. For example, the Society for the Study of Social Biology has aims of 'furthering knowledge about biological and socio-cultural forces which affect the composition and structure of human populations'. Some social biologists continue to seek correlations between disease and race, and such work can be subject to the limitations which Cooper discusses in the following chapter. In addition there are many discordant views in borderline subjects such as social biology and many sociologists and anthropologists are not united in their assessment of biology [29]. However, at this point, it is appropriate to discuss the evolution of medical geography as another borderline discipline, and to illustrate the development of geographical interest in the subject matter of the book.

MEDICAL GEOGRAPHY AND THE STUDY OF HEALTH AND HEALTH
CARE

Medical geography has a long history of researching
both disease ecology and health care provision and
planning [30-36]. Nevertheless, whilst it has tended
to focus on the spatial-geographical aspects of
disease and health care, geographers have generally
been very appreciative amongst social scientists of
the need to study a wide range of variables in these
and related topics. Some of the first contemporary
geographical studies of health and health care were
carried out under the auspices of the Chicago
Regional Hospital study from the mid-1960s [37,38].
This broad-ranging project and subsequent research
identified important prejudicial features of health
services such as the predilection of some parts of
the service to serve only people of certain race,
income or religion. The problems of access to
health care for black patients have been highlighted
in these and many other studies in the United
States [39-41]. The ultimate in spatial proximity
but social distance has also been identified when
black neighbourhoods in urban transitional zones are
situated very close to central business district
physicians' offices. Most of the black residents
would be unable to afford these central city
physicians' services and, therefore, have often had
to find their way to more distant clinics and to
hospital emergency departments. In this way,
social barriers can lead to longer than necessary
journeys for care and more general spatial
disadvantages have long been identified as cause
for concern in medical geography research.
Subsequently, more general interest has developed
with social and spatial justice. This has arisen
in part from the 'welfare approach' in human
geography: Smith summarises this by posing the
question who gets what, when and where: the
questions how and at what cost and of what quality
may also be added [42]. The criteria of spatial
justice may be applied to analyse settings in which
there is unequal physical distribution and
accessibility to a range of services or
opportunities, of which health care is but one.
Spatial as well as social injustice may be explicit
in a system as in apartheid [43] or it can arise
from the distributional inequalities inherent in
capitalist space economies and the unequal access to
resources deriving from it, as facilities generally

locate in response to economic forces and not to overt need.

How have geographers developed the concept of social, spatial and territorial justice with regard to health and health care? Apart from documenting obvious differences in levels of health between groups (social classes or ethnic groups, perhaps), geographers have attempted to feed into health care policy to enhance accessibility and utilisation of services [44]. Knox, for example, has called for positive discrimination in public policy towards resource allocation [45] and Rathwell discusses the identification of 'special care groups' who may become the 'targets' for certain policies [46]. Some approaches may hinge on defining zones in which policies may be directed - the so-called areal approach - or may apply to special groups in two populations. Clearly, in terms of enhancing the health and health care of ethnic minorities, both approaches might have some validity. At a general level, it has been noted that there are spatial concentrations of ethnic minorities in certain parts of some cities; however, not all residents in these areas will be equally disadvantaged so a blanket areal approach may not be effective [47,48]. After the delineation of target or policy areas (or even instead of it), it may be desirable to define special care groups towards whom policies may be directed. We take up the discussion of the nature of some policies which might be effective in this regard in the concluding chapter.

This links with a relatively new theme in human geography in which research is being directed towards disadvantaged consumers. These may often be the members of ethnic minorities but they may involve other disadvantaged groups also. Herbert and Thomas [49] and Joseph and Phillips [50] discuss the notion that some sections of communities may be less well able to use health services than others, which stems from findings in other spheres of consumer research. Disadvantaged consumers may be the lowest social classes, elderly or disabled persons, or members of ethnic minorities who are restricted to whatever services exist locally because of a combination of low incomes and constraints on personal mobility. In effect, the choice and selectivity which other people have are denied to disadvantaged consumers. With regard to the use of health services provided by a majority from a different group, members of ethnic minorities may be subjected to additional disadvantages. For

11

example,   there may be linguistic barriers which may
hinder   (or   even   prevent)   communication between
patient   and   professional;   treatments   may be
perceived to be inappropriate or some ailments may
not even be recognised as such by the system.
     It is easy to envisage this type of consumer
disadvantage with regard to health care. Members of
some Asian communities may, for instance, prefer to
use traditional healers or traditional medicines and
there is an increasing number of hakims and vaids in
many western countries, particularly Britain [51].
These physicians practise, respectively, the unani
and ayurvedic medicine systems of the Indian sub-
continent.   However,   their   services   are not
generally available or provided by national health
services, or covered by health insurance, and they
are not universally accessible to persons who might
wish to consult them. Therefore, a type of
disadvantage is clearly reflected in the lack of
perceived appropriate care which would be selected
by choice.   This might have distinct geographical
features relating to the distribution of traditional
practitioners in relation to minority groups. It
also has important policy implications relating to
the need for much greater flexibility on the part of
the service to provide appropriate types of care
which might not be generally desired by the majority
of the population.
     Many Asians feel that a hakim or vaid is likely
to respond to them more sympathetically than do most
allopathic doctors, including those of south Asian
origins.   In addition, their remedies are believed
to be more efficacious for certain conditions.
Nevertheless the medical establishment hardly
recognises the type of community service such
traditional practitioners can provide to ethnic
groups. As a result, they do not receive official
recognition and support which would enable them to
extend their services.   This illustrates consumer
disadvantage in the lack of provision for
appropriate care from minority groups.   It is,
however, pertinent to point out that even in some
countries where traditional medicine flourishes, it
may not receive official recognition or financial
support from the state.   Ironically, this can be
true in some Third World countries where the
existence of traditional medicine may be felt to
reflect 'backwardness' [52].
     Medical geographers are interested in
researching the health circumstances of many
minority groups, and as editors, we are aware that

most chapters do reflect a concern for minorities.
The main exception is Fincham's case study which
portrays the situation in South Africa of a majority
but one for whom lack of political and economic
power is formalised and institutionalised. His
paper highlights the appalling conditions of many
living under apartheid whose voice is in effect
vastly less than that of their minority government.
The other chapters discuss societies which consider
themselves avowedly to be equal; indeed, racial
discrimintion is illegal in them although, as a
number of authors show, disadvantages can flourish
even when equal opportunities purport to exist.

THE STRUCTURE OF THE BOOK

The book has been organised in two main parts. The
first considers definitional matters, some almost of
a theoretical nature. Richard Cooper's chapter has
developed from a key 'position paper' in the
conference and provides a broad overview about
ethnicity, race and disease, placing in historical
context the various genetic, social and
environmental aetiologies which have been postulated
from time to time to explain the incidence of
disease. He then proceeds to outline the history
of the anti-racist movement mainly in the United
States tracing its political origins and current
status.
      Ranjit Bandaranyake's paper in this section
is also a contribution from a physician, this time
one working as an epidemiologist in Britain. His
focus is on the differences in diseases within
populations, in this instance subdivided according
to ethnic backgrounds. He also highlights disease
incidence rates at the local scale of Bradford
Health District where the prevalence of some
conditions is much higher among ethnic groups than
in the white population although for other
conditions, prevalence is lower. Nevertheless, all
these differential incidence rates can cause concern
in terms of social justice and equality of life-
chances. It is apposite that this paper follows Dr.
Cooper's since readers will have been reminded that
in the absence of any genetic or biological
explanations for these differences in incidence
rates, the facts must indicate enormous disparities
and inequalities on a range of social and economic
factors in which the ethnic groups are
disadvantaged. Dr. Bandaranayake concludes by

13

indicating the potential for collaborative links for
sharing data between the health services and local
authorities, the establishment of integrated
information systems being of benefit to all parties.
    The third paper of the introductory section, by
Maggie Pearson, asks a fundamental question about
ethnic health studies: whether they are of true
scientific value and of potential help to ethnic
groups or whether they are 'subtle oppressive
measures' which might have the rather reactionary
effect of containing or defusing justifiable black
dissent. This question is, of course, very
difficult to answer and the editors are aware that
this book might be subject to such criticism. The
defence is that the intention is certainly to
provide practical policy strategies based on the
empirical evidence presented but readers have to
make up their own minds whether this is achieved or
even advisable. This paper puts the debate, the
strengths and weaknesses of the 'race relations
business' into stark perspective and certainly
indicates that an important question mark hangs over
much work in the health and related fields.
    Part Two of the book provides a series of
empirical and policy-oriented articles on health and
health care for ethnic groups. The intention is to
develop something of a bridge between theory and
practice and the authors cover a small but important
range of countries. Marianne Lauridsen discusses
the relatively new phenomenon of ethnic minorities
in Denmark and the need for sensitive provision of
health care in a country with a high overall
standard of living but where the small ethnic
minorities seem to be relatively disadvantaged on a
number of indices. The Danish policy of
integration of minorities but with state support for
providing appropriate health care and some of the
responsibilites being devolved onto the ethnic
groups, provides an interesting practical model
which may be of relevance for other countries.
    The paper by Professor Griffiths and co-authors
from Michigan takes a more statistically oriented
approach to the analysis of hospital utilisation
rates by black and white groups. This detailed
paper provides something of a contrast to others in
the book in that the results suggest some lessening
of inequalities in access to, and use of, hospitals
in Michigan when morbidity and use rates are taken
into account. To an extent this is encouraging but
blacks do use hospitals more than whites but not
when their extra need is taken into account.

14

Ethnicity and Health: Introduction and Definitions

Robert Fincham paints a much bleaker picture with
regard to nutritional status of black communities in
the Eastern Cape, South Africa. Based on extensive
local research, severe levels of malnutrition are
identified and some possible methods of intervention
to improve this picture are suggested, with the
implicit recognition that any attempts are at
present likely to have to be within the existing
political and economic framework, a limiting but
realistic observation perhaps.
     The remaining papers in Part Two are based
largely in a British context although John Giggs for
example provides a brief review of the international
literature about ethnic status and mental illness.
He discusses the incidence of schizophrenia amongst
ethnic groups in Nottingham, finding a complex
picture of distribution and occurrence. An
interesting example is provided of the use of
geographical methodology to investigate the
distribution of a specific form of mental illness
which could valuably be applied in other intra-urban
settings. This paper is usefully complemented by
another intra-urban study, this time of the
availability and use of primary health care services
in the West Midlands. Mark Johnson, a medical
geographer based at the Centre for Research on
Ethnic Relations in the University of Warwick,
provides as he says not a definitive statement on
the use of health services by ethnic minorities but
a picture of the variations in usage of services
amongst groups and in different locations. Contrary
to many existing views, he suggests that ethnic
minorities do not seem to make excessive or
unreasonable demands on the curative services and
they also display positive attitudes to preventive
services. Nevertheless, he reminds readers of the
important factor that disadvantage can exist in the
health services as in many other spheres of life and
he poses important questions regarding the quality
of professional care which may be provided for some
groups. It is up to professionals to improve the
delivery of the service: it is not necessarily up
to consumers to alter their needs or demands.
     Finally, Jenny Donovan's paper provides
stimulus for researchers in this general area. She
draws particular attention to the shortcomings of
research into 'unusual' ailments which may afflict
ethnic minorities, highlighting the dangers of
classifying all ethnic group members as 'problems'
as discussed previously. She provides a useful
study of how variables related to religion, work,

racism, expected remedies and the like can influence what black people feel about their health and the health services. Whilst definitive answers are not provided, the nature of individuals' self-perception and expections are illustrated and this gives a humanising insight which is arguably lacking in some other papers in the book. The respondents show through, discussing their own ideas about health and health services; for once, a detailed 'depersonalised' statistical approach is avoided.

POLICY APPLICATIONS: POSITIVE ACTION OR PAPERING THE CRACKS?

The contributors to this book illustrate that many people within and outside health services in a number of countries are very concerned about the unresponsiveness of society and health services to ethnic needs. We hope that this collection will provide some impetus and encouragement at the personal and policy level to improve this situation.

In our final chapter we explore more fully the possible policy implications of some of the papers and try to draw some general conclusions from the range of work within the book. We would at this juncture like to state that, as McNaught suggests [53] although the assessment is largely negative of many current and past intitiatives to improve the provision, accessibility and appropriateness of health care for ethnic groups, this must not be taken to indicate that no practical progress may be achieved in the future. We must learn from our mistakes and shortcomings.

In particular, perhaps, we might note that in virtually all the countries covered in this book with the exception of South Africa, discriminative behaviour towards people on the grounds of race or ethnicity is prohibited in law. However, the most carefully encoded laws and race relations policies cannot be effective unless there is good will but even this in itself is not sufficient. There has to be some clear mechanisms of achieving improvement; a legal framework and a willing population can help but positive policies form the only way of implementing reform. Perhaps this book may help the growth and development of those elements of nascent frameworks that exist at present.

16

However, many aspects of policy are essentially status quo and may be designed to mollify disadvantaged groups or individuals without altering or removing the fundamental causes of disadvantage. If policies are designed only to 'paper over the cracks' in a social system rather than redesigning and rebuilding the structure on a sounder basis, then policy may be at best partially successful and, at worst, merely prolong an inequitable situation. The suggestions which come through in a number of the chapters and those which we provide in our conclusions must be evaluated in the light of this knowledge.

REFERENCES

1. Gobineau, A. De (1915) Racial inequality is not the result of institutions, reprinted in J. Stone, (ed) Race, Ethnicity and Social Change, Duxbury Press, Massachusetts, 1977, pp. 10-13, Essai sur L'Inegalite de Race Humaines appeared first in 1853
2. Zubaida, S. (ed) (1970) Race and Racialism, Tavistock, London
3. UNESCO (1975) Race, Science and Society, Columbia University Press, New York
4. Stone, J. (ed) (1977) Race, Ethnicity and Social Change, Duxbury Press, Massachusetts, p. xi
5. Bujra, J.(1983) Cultural and Social Diversity: a Third World in the Making in U204, Third World Studies, The Making of the Third World, Block 2, Part A, pp. 9, The Open University Press, Milton Keynes
6. Ibid.
7. Donovan, J. (1984) Ethnicity and health: a research reveiw, Social Science and Medicine, Vol. 19, pp. 663-670
8. Husband, C. (ed) (1982) 'Race' in Britain: Continuity and Change, Hutchinson, London, pp. 16
9. Ahmed, S. (1984) 'Second generation immigrant' is a complete distortion of English, Social Work Today, Vol. 16, 10 September, pp. 12-13
10. Donovan, J. (1984) op. cit.
11. Smith, D.J. (1976) The Facts of Racial Disadvantage, Vol. XLII, Broadsheet No. 560, Political and Economic Planning, London

12. Donovan, J. (1984) op. cit.
13. Ibid.
14. McNaught, A. (1984) Race and Health Care in the United Kingdom, Centre for Health Service Management Studies, Polytechnic of the South Bank, London
15. Smith, D.J. (1976) op. cit.
16. Community Relations Commission (1977) Urban Deprivation, Racial Inequality and Social Policy, H.M.S.O., London
17. Khan, V.S. (ed) (1979) Minority Families in Britain, Macmillan, London
18. Field, S. (1984) The Attitudes of Ethnic Minorities, Home Office Research Study, No. 80, H.M.S.O., London
19. Littlewood, R. and Lipsedge, M. (1982) Aliens and Alienists: Ethnic Minorities and Psychiatry, Penguin, Harmondsworth
20. Rack, P. (1982) Race, Culture and Mental Disorder, Tavistock, London
21. Johnson, M.R.D. (1983) Race and Health: a Select Bibliography, SSRC Research Unit on Ethnic Relations, University of Aston, Birmingham
22. Harwood, A. (ed) (1981) Ethnicity and Medical Care, Harvard University Press, Cambridge
23. Bullough, V. and Bullough, B. (1982) Health Care for the Other Americans, Second Edition, Appleton-Century-Crofts, Connecticut
24. Blakemore, K. (1982) Health and illness among the elderly of minority ethnic groups living in Birmingham: some new findings, Health Trends, Vol. 14, pp. 69-72
25. McNeedy, R.L. and Colen, J.L. (eds) (1983) Aging in Minority Groups, Sage Publications, Beverly Hills, California
26. MacCormack, C. (1980) Health care problems of ethnic minority groups, MIMS Magazine, 15 July, pp. 53-60
27. Wilkes, R. (1985) Social Work With Undervalued Groups, Tavistock, London
28. Torkington, N.P.K. (1983) The Racial Politics of Health - a Liverpool Profile, Merseyside Area Profile Group, Department of Sociology, University of Liverpool, Liverpool

29. Wiegle,   T.C.   (ed.)   (1982)   Biology and the
     Social   Sciences: an   Emerging Evolution
     Westview Press, Boulder, Colorado
30. Shannon,   G.W. and Dever, G.E.A. (1974)   Health
     Care   Delivery: Spatial   Perspectives,
     McGraw-Hill, New York
31. Learmonth,   A.T.A. (1978)   Patterns of Disease
     and Hunger, David and Charles, Newton
     Abbot
32. Pyle, G.F.   (1979) Applied Medical Geography,
     Wiley, New York
33. Phillips,   D.R. (1981)   Contemporary Issues in
     the Geography of Health Care, Geo Books,
     Norwich
34. McGlashan,   N.D. and Blunden, J. (eds) (1983)
     Geographical Aspects of Health, Academic
     Press, London
35. Eyles,   J. and Woods, K.J. (1983)   The Social
     Geography of Medicine and Health, Croom
     Helm, London
36. Joseph,   A.E.   and   Phillips,   D.R. (1984)
     Accessibility   and   Utilization:
     Geographical Perspectives on Health Care
     Delivery, Harper and Row, London
37. Morrill,   R.L.   and Earickson, R.J. (1968)
     Variations in the Character and Use
     of Hospital Services, Health Services
     Research, pp. 224-238
38. Earickson, R.J. (1970) The spatial behavior of
     hospital   patients,   Department   of
     Geography   Research Paper No.   124,
     University of Chicago
39. Vise,   P. de (1973) Misused and misplaced
     hospitals and doctors, Commission on
     College Geography Resource Paper 22,
     Association of American Geographers,
     Washington
40. Shannon,   G.W. and Dever, G.E.A. (1974) op.
     cit.
41. Shannon,   G.W., Spurlock, C.W. and Bashshur,
     R.L. (1975) The search for health
     care, and exploration of urban black
     behavior, Proceedings of the Association
     of American Geographers, Vol. 7, pp. 215-
     221
42. Smith, D.M. (1974) Who gets what where and how:
     a welfare focus for human geography,
     Geography, Vol. 59, pp. 289-297
43. Smith, D.M. (1977) Human Geography: a Welfare
     Approach, Edward Arnold, London

44. Joseph,   A.E.   and   Phillips,   D.R. (1984) op. cit.
45. Knox, P.L.   (1979)   Medical   deprivation,   area deprivation   and   public   policy,   Social Science and Medicine, vol. 13D, pp. 11-121
46. Rathwell, T. (1984) General practice, ethnicity and   health   services   delivery,   Social Science   and   Medicine,   vol. 19, pp. 123-130
47. Smith,   D.M.   (1979)   The   identification of problems   in   cities: the application of social   indicators,   in D T Herbert and D M Smith   (eds) Social Problems and the City, Oxford   University   Press, Oxford, pp. 13-32
48. Phillips, D.R. (1981) op. cit.
49. Herbert,   D.T.   and   Thomas, C.J. (1982) Urban Geography: a   First   Approach,   Wiley, Chichester
50. Joseph,   A.E.   and   Phillips,   D.R. (1984) op. cit.
51. Ballard,   R.   (1979)   Ethnic Minorities and the Social   Service,   in V S Khan (ed) Minority Families   in   Britain,   Macmillan, London, pp. 147-164
52. Kikhela,   N.,   Bibeau,   G. and Corin, E. (1981) Africa's   two medical systems: options for planners,   World Health Forum, Vol. 2, pp. 96-99
53. McNaught, A. (1984) op. cit.

Chapter 2

RACE, DISEASE AND HEALTH

Richard Cooper

INTRODUCTION

Race is a powerful determinant of health. In
virtually every multi-racial society consistent
patterns of differential mortality have been
described. Most of the international variation in
health indices likewise follow racial lines.
Although marked improvement has been observed for
all racial groups over this century, the fundamental
relative differences in health status persist.
    There is no evidence that a major proportion of
the observed racial differentials in health can be
explained in population genetics. Environmental
forces, namely social conditions, are the root
cause. Racial inequality in health is a basic
feature of social stratification in today's world;
it reflects the underlying class structure of
capitalism and calls into question the legitimacy of
a social system which produces such grossly unequal
life chances. At the same time, the forces which
lead to racial differentials play a fundamental role
in determining health patterns for the rest of
society. This is true for the determination of
differentials across class, sex, age and geographic
region, as well as the over-all disease pattern.
Both these considerations - bad health for the
oppressed racial group, per se, and the effect of
racism on the health of society as a whole - argue
for the central importance of race in the study of
contemporary public health problems.
    Conventional approaches to the health problems
of oppressed and exploited racial groups have
suffered from a variety of weaknesses. Although
explanations based on biological determinism (that
is, genetics) no longer enjoy consensus support in
most scientifc disciplines, they exert grossly
disproportionate influence in public health and
continue to mould popular wisdom. By the same
token, the analysis which 'controls for socio-
economic conditions' entirely misses the point about
race; it is or can be construed as a socio-economic

21

category. In   the   search   for   solutions the
missionary   vision   of   the   era   of imperialist
expansion   has   been   reshaped   into   liberal and
moralistic social engineering.   Likewise, raising
the alarm among the majority that the presence of an
unhealthy race in their midst poses a great threat
from   contagion   is   an   insufficient   basis for
generating a social movement to cure the root
cause.
        The existence of important racial differentials
in disease demonstrates that society is destroying
health.   The   effect   of   these   destructive forces
cannot   be   limited   to   the   most   oppressed racial
group;   the burden must be borne in some measure by
all.   The mechanism of disease spread may be one of
spill-over,   or   shared exposure, as in a relatively
integrated   society   like   the United States (US) or
mutual   destruction through the opposites of surfeit
and   starvation, as in South Africa. The disruptive
forces   generated   by racism further contribute to a
lowering   of   the level of health care services. As
captured   dramatically   in   Marx's   metaphor   about
British   rule   in   India,   an   unequal yet universal
sacrifice   of   health   is   the   price paid to set in
motion   the   productive   machinery   in   societies
stratified by race and class.
        Based   on   the perspective outlined above, this
paper will discuss the following topics: first, the
concept   of   race;   second,   racism   as   a class
question;   thirdly,   racial differentials in health
within the United States; fourthly, race and health
in   an   international   perspective;   fifthly, racism
and health care services and, lastly, the resurgence
of racism today.

THE CONCEPT OF RACE

Race and Biology: an Historical view
The meaning of race has been vigorously debated
since   the   concept   was   first introduced some   200
years ago [1-6].   Although properly the concern of
anthropologists, the pervasive impact of the concept
of   race   has   made   this   question   one of everyday
importance   for   all   social   scientists.   Indeed,
coming   to   terms   with   the   problem   of race is an
essential   requirement   for   anyone   who wants to be
more   than   a   victim   of the political forces which
shape   today's   world.   A   brief   review   of these
historical   questions   is   necessary   to   provide a
context for the discussion of race and health.

22

The concept of race as applied to man was first introduced into the literature of biology by Buffon in 1749 [7]. It was explicitly regarded as an arbitrary classfication, serving only as a convenient label not a definable scientific entity. From the point of view of the biologist, the concept of race is an attempt to extend the taxonomic classification below the level of species. It shares the inherent weaknesses of the Linnaen system, while introducing unique problems of its own. Taxonomy is useful for two separate, but inter-related, reasons: firstly it helps the understanding of evolution; and secondly it provides a framework for examining present variation in plants and animals. Yet no zoological classification is absolute [8-10]. As Watts points out, "from an evolutionary point of view taxonomy is arbitrary and static. Forcing the results of the dynamic and multiplex process of evolution into a simple two-dimensional set of pigeon-holes cannot be done without losing information" [11]. For most biologists use of race results in a net loss of information.

If consensus is any measure, defining the races of man has never been successfully accomplished [12-16]. It is important to emphasise that what is at stake here is not the possibility of designating groups of people that differ in some way. Human variation is self-evident; the existence of definable groups, or races, is not. The scientific purpose of the concept of race is therefore to give meaning to human variation, not merely to point out one or another aspect of that variation [17]. It goes without saying that race must at the same time delineate importance and consistent genetic differences; it implies that a 'package' of different genes, all of which ideally should be known, exist between groups. Why is it that on both counts historical efforts to use the race concept scientifically have ended in monumental failure?

First, geographic variation in gene frequency is mainly quantitative, or clinical in nature. From Europe eastward across the Asian land-mass populations merge into one another. Circular phenomena also occur; that is, moving in one direction gene frequencies gradually change, until arriving back at the point of origin where a sharp break may be observed. The problem of indistinct borders for racial groups might be solved by accepting several large races, say two to five.

However, the number of non-classifiable groups will be great. The other extreme would be to reduce each population or 'ethnic group' to a separate category. This is essentially the process of naming, not classifying, and is the approach taken by Dobzhansky et al [18].

Second, human variation is primarily discordant, rather than concordant. That is, while two groups may be similar in skin colour, they differ in other important features, such as height, blood type, and facial features. To classify on the basis of skin colour arbitrarily assigns primary importance to that characteristic, and forces all others to be ignored. Is there any reason to believe that variations in skin colour subsume all, or any, biologically important human variations? The Masai, pygmies of the African rain forest, inhabitants of southern India, Australian aborigines, and natives of the Amazon delta are all dark skinned; are they members of the same race? Skin colour in these groups probably reflects a common history of exposure to ultraviolet radiation, not a common racial origin.

No discrete 'package' of gene differences has ever been described between two races, only relative frequencies of one or another trait. Yet one might ask, is it not common practice in medicine and biology to divide a continuous distribution into discrete categories? Haemoglobin, blood pressure, and body mass index are all skewed normal distributions; yet one accepts the validity of the concepts of anaemia, hypertension and obesity. For pathological conditions (such as hypertension) one has objective criteria (association with morbid sequels), while for racial traits no such external reference system exists. The unusual case, like sickle cell anaemia, can be easily handled on its own merit without reference to a malfitting racial category. Just as single-gene abnormalities are recognised to be different from most diseases which require complication gene-environment interaction, consistent difference in one gene between populations is rare and cannot express anything more than a miniscule portion of the total potential variation.

A single trait, such as skin colour, is not an adequate basis for characterising human diversity. Variation in a single gene, like that for sickle cell, does not imply that populations which vary in that gene will vary in important ways from any other health condition. Transferring racial

susceptibility from, say, sickle cell anaemia to
cancer, is an unjustified assumption. Discordant
variation implies that unless two conditions can be
shown to be linked they should be assumed to be
independent. Most public health analysis based on
racial categories adopts this false analogy – that a
'package' of genetic differences exists - and is
therefore fatally flawed.

Even if one could classify groups of people
usefully by race little would have been accomplished
from the point of view of the anthropologist.
"Races as genetic groups can only really be
understood in terms of the process by which they
originated" [19]. Coon argued that the five races
of man represent separate origins of the human
species, with independent evolutionary
histories [20]. This position has been widely
discredited. The search for 'pure' races is a
false hope [21,22]. One does not have a history of
man's wandering, nor will it ever be forthcoming.
"It is an error to believe that races are things
whose separate evolutionary development may be
traced" [23]. Although this limitation may be fatal
for the anthropologist, it could still be argued
that the epidemiologist needs a system which gives
broad categories of gene distribution [24]. The
epidemiologist presumably is not very interested in
the origin of genes, wishing to know of their
present distribution, and therefore does not need to
know anything about the 'process by which they
originated' to understand 'races as genetic groups'.
Again there is a false analogy applicable: race is
only potentially useful because it might 'explain'
something about evolution. Man's health problems
today are not in any major way a result of his
evolutionary history, in the physical sense; it is
cultural history which has produced the human
disease burden. The genetic evolutionary baggage
purportedly contained in the concept of race is
therefore of no interest to the epidemiologist
either, except in the rarest cases. The rare cases
– for example, sickle cell in some blacks and skin
cancer in white Australians – cannot justify the
dominant role given genetic explanation of between-
race disease variation.

Despite these criticisms the biological
concept of race is still used routinely today by
many biologists and anthropologists [25-27]. Among
its most prominent supporters has been Theodosius
Dobzhansky, who wrote in 1962 "anthropologists are
confronted with a diversity of human beings . . .

Figure 2.1:   Ratio of Death Rates from all Causes,
Nonwhite: White, Age-Specific, Males, Ages 5-75,
1960-1980

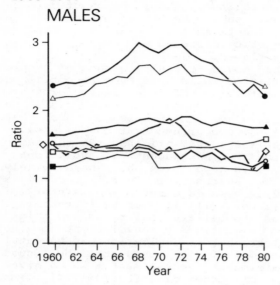

Figure 2.2:   Ratio of Death Rates from all Causes,
Nonwhite,:   White, Age-Specific, Females, Ages 5-75,
1960-1980

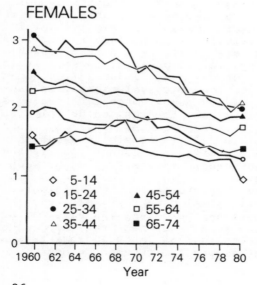

Race is the subject of scientific study and analysis simply because it is a fact of nature" [28]. While acknowledging the views of critics, this position was maintained in the most recent edition of his influential textbook on evolution [29]. It is argued that "races, species, genera, and other categories are needed above all for the pragmatic purpose of communication" [30], yet a very limited defence for continued use of the category is offered. Race is returned to the status proposed by Buffon, a label of pure convenience. Thus, there may be 'European' and 'African' races on one occasion, and on another 'Nordics, Alpines, Mediterraneans, Armeniods' [31]. Accepting this definition it is hard to disagree with an earlier conclusion by these same authors: "Saying that a population is of such-and-such geographic origin is good enough" [32].

To name various population groups for the sake of comparing gene frequencies is not the same as creating a classification of homo sapiens based on race. The 'name' process in effect denies the assumption that races have a structural relationship to each other, because of evolution, and that each category has systematic differences in a block or package of genes. Thus use of the racial category implies that the groups are different in characteristics other than the primary one being compared. Otherwise, why not specify precisely the population and the trait? It is this assumption of consistent differences in traits which is the essential failure of the concept of race.

One final question must be addressed: How important is the potential racial variation? Glass has suggested that the number of gene differences between, say a West African and a Native of Denmark, may be very small indeed. He estimates that the 'white race' differs characteristically - that is, on a population basis - by no more than six pairs of genes from the black [33]. While others consider this estimate low, it serves to place this question in its proper context [34]. Typical variations within a population are in orders of magnitude. Given the overall magnitude of potential variation, two persons of the same race could vary by thousands of genes. Lewontin has estimated that diversity between individuals in a population accounts for 85 per cent of the total species variation, diversity within race accounts for 8.3 per cent, and between-race diversity contributesonly 6.3 per cent [35]. While consistent differences, such as skin colour, may tell us more about adaptive change than random, white-population, variation, they will be overwhelmed by the weight of similarity when examining man as a species. More recent consideration of 'Haldane's dilemma' suggests that systematic variation between populations may be primarily due to genetic drift, rather than adaptation, thereby eliminating even the possible significance of racial differences from an evolutionary point of view [36]. Accordingly, there is no evidence, that racial variation in disease is in any but the most trivial way genetic in origin. Different human populations exposed to similar environments are much more alike than different in their disease rates.

The Race Concept and Public Health

The concept of race is prominent in public health and medicine. The classic anthropological concept of race is used almost exclusively - where the race label identifies a set (package, block) of important genetic differences, however ill-defined. The obscure phenotypic variations, based on observations from small numbers of individuals with totally unknown genetic resemblance, are ascribed to 'racial differences' [37]. True genetic markers are rarely used and the relationship between genotype and phenotype is almost universally ignored. A strong hereditarian bias also exists in medicine, independent of the question of race.

Racial differentials in virtually all diseases have been attributed to genetic factors. Common infectious diseases are no exception. Classic studies on rheumatic fever in the last century from England clearly demonstrated the risk associated with poverty and crowding [38]. Newsholme, based on a careful review of this data, concluded in 1895 that "the influence of heredity has been exaggerated" and "as to race there is no evidence" [39]. Nonetheless, in the United States it was considered that rheumatic fever was a disease to which the Irish were racially susceptible and that it was linked to genes for red hair [40]. As the Irish became more prosperous the disease disappeared, to recur in black migrants from the rural South in urban centres [41].

What is the central meaning of the concept of race as applied to public health? In public health and medical work race is virtually never defined, that is, specific gene frequencies are rarely measured and the criteria for assignment to one or another race are not stated. In fact, all humans, in terms of their susceptibility to all but the rarest of diseases, are genetically similar. Systematic variation in susceptibility has not been shown to fall along racial lines for any common disease. Racial differences reflect different social environments, not different genes, even where two groups live side by side, such as black and whites in the US. <u>Race does not mark in any important way for genetic traits, rather it demonstrates beyond question the paramount role of social causes</u>.

Blacks in the US have age-sex-specific mortality ratios which are 23 to 300 per cent higher than whites. These ratios are likewise highly mobile over time (Figures 2.1 and 2.2). How can they be genetic? Age-adjusted death rates for blacks were 37 per cent higher than for whites in the US in 1977. The most common fatal illness for which we have a clear-cut racial/genetic explanation is sickle cell disease. In 1977, there were 80,000 excess black deaths compared to white; 277 black deaths were coded to hemoglobinopathies, or 0.3 per cent of the total excess. An explanation for the rest of the excess mortality must be sought in social causes.

In summary, race is a social concept and as such has no specific biological meaning. It lives on today on the fringes of science in blatant contradiction to all that is known from the study of human variation. It is more than the 'phlogiston' of our time [42]. Unlike phlogiston it has not been expunged from scientific discourse by reasoned arguments or well-marshalled facts. The availability of a correct explanation eventually defeated phlogiston because it opened the door for progress in physical science. Capitalism needed the physical sciences; it decidedly does not need social equality. Racism has not been defeated because it continues to hold the key to further 'progress' within the social system. Race provides an essential basis for the continued accumulation of capital and its concentration in fewer hands. A reflection of the social world, and not the natural world, the race concept will not be expunged until that social world is changed. All important group variation in disease can be adequately described while totally disregarding concerns about between-population genetic factors. The concept of race, as currently used, has only served to obscure this fact. It has thereby greatly hindered any understanding of geographic pathology and, instead, serves only to help justify racial inequality in health.

RACE AS A CLASS QUESTION

Slavery and the Origins of Racism
If the concept of race has no legitimate scientific claim to existence, why has it remained such a vital part of cultural experience? Unlike out-moded concepts of evolution or the solar system, the vast majority of people in society, including no doubt most scientists, firmly believe that races do exist; by the same token, the race concept retains a prominent role in the explanation of disease variation. How else could the likes of Burt, Coon and E.O. Wilson, rise to positions of great importance by simply advocating questionable theories of genetic superiority? Clearly the history of race transcends any strict scientific analysis. It must fulfil an important social need.

In human society popular acceptance of the social order requires an ideology. 'The great chain of being' entitled the kings and their minions to privilege and power. In that social environment Galileo and Darwin found more than scientific opposition to their new theories. The class structure of capitalism likewise requires ideological assumptions to justify its existence. In addition to inalienable social privilege based on ownership of property, people in society are highly stratified by class, race, sex, age and nationality. Races do very much exist in society. Bourgeois science assumes the task of making that existence appear natural. Race can therefore only be understood as a social question, as a product of the class structure of society. Given the current competitive structure of the world-wide capitalist economy, racism is essential to the maintenance of the status quo; without it, present levels of profitability could not be maintained and restructuring of the world markets would occur.

Boyd argues that although early societies had many forms of class and caste "the concept of race, as an immutable physical entity as we now know it, probably did not exist" [43]. Montague has been one of the more prominent exponents of the idea that the emergence of the African slave trade, the key to the development of European capitalism in the 17th and 18th century, led to invention of the modern concept of race [44]. While the slave trade was crucial in the origin of racism, a second development of this historical era had a more enduring effect on capitalist society.

It was in America that the impact of slavery was felt most directly. The long-term need of a growing multi-racial society demanded the invention of institutional racism.

> The first Africans in Virginia, most historians agree, were classified as indentured servants. The status of 'slave' simply did not exist. The low condition to which indentured servants were subjected signalled a form of labour organisation unique to the New World. It was not possible to observe the European forms of labour organisation and relations in a context where land was widely available and opportunities generally open. The large fortunes to be made from the cultivation of tobacco would simply not have been possible without forced servitude.
>
> It was into this world that Africans were brought in 1619. At first they were treated little differently from indentured servants, except perhaps in the length of their service. Details are obscure, but it appears that while some Africans served their entire lives, others earned freedom, at least in the period before 1660. Only after 1650 did laws and social practices distinguishing black workers from whites begin to appear in Virginia. [45]

With the arrival of greater numbers of white workers, and the survival of many blacks beyond the period of servitude, class conflict began to develop in the young colonies. Anti-black racism served to unite the white colonials and diffuse antagonisms between rich and poor classes. Slavery, and its identification exclusively with people of colour, thus served two purposes: it provided a tractable work force for the plantation economy as well as a unifying impetus to white society. The former purpose served US capitalism well for the first two hundred years of its existence; the latter has done so equally well for the last hundred [46-50].

In contemporary capitalist society, racism
serves a dual, inter-related function. In the
economic sphere, racism increases the profitability
of capital in two ways: first by directly lowering
the wage rate for the oppressed group and, secondly,
by the divisive power of racial divisions which
weaken the working class as a whole so wages for the
majority, or 'non-oppressed' racial groups, can be
lowered as well. The first of those two mechanisms
will be referred to as 'super-exploitation' and the
second as the 'class effect of racism'. In the
political sphere racism provides a coherent ideology
which binds the working class majority to the power
structure, as it did in colonial Virginia.

History of the anti-Racist Movement
The left-wing movement, either through its own
efforts or by stimulating a liberal response, has
been the main social force which has advanced the
cause of anti-racism over the last century [51-54].
Marx provided one of the first clear formulations of
the class perspective on racism: "Labour in the
white skin will never be free while it is branded in
the black". Although the development of a
scientific understanding has been slow, the class
orientation of the communist movement led the
struggle against fascism and the extreme forms of
racial supremacy which developed during World War
II, both in Europe and in Asia. In the US the
left-wing movement in general played a key role in
the fight for unionisation of black workers and
civil rights [55-57]. Particularly important were
the anti-lynching campaigns of the US Communist
Party and the industrial unions [58].

Liberal approaches to racism have been
predicated on two assumptions. First, liberals
assume without question that the constitutions of
modern capitalist states guarantee equal rights –
they need only be realised in practice. Second,
they argue that racism has been diminishing over the
long-term, and will presumably disappear with time.
Chief academic spokesman of the liberal position in
the early 1940s was Gunnar Myrdal. In his
influential book, <u>An American Dilemma</u>, he wrote:

Negroes are discriminated against in practically all spheres of life, but in their fight for equal opportunity they have on their side the law of the land and the religion of the nation. No social Utopia can compete with the promises of the American Constitution and with the American Creed which it embodies . . . Merely by giving him the solemn promise of equality and liberty, American society has tied the Negroes' faith to itself. [59]

The anti-racist movement in the US continued to make progress in the 1950s and 1960s. This period also led to a resurgence of the attack on the race concept by anthropologists and other liberal academics, as well as fairly widespread political and social reforms. The rhetoric of complete equality became even sharper as the government became actively involved in efforts to reduce the impact of racism. While change did occur over this period, there was nothing approaching a fundamental restructuring of social relations and the gains were more symbolic and political. The appearance of change, rather than economic progress, thereby became the hallmark of liberal programmes. Attention was given to anti-racist demands only to prevent the hope of eventual equality from losing all basis in reality.

Whatever judgement one makes on the potential of the liberal programme to offer real solutions, its theoretical formulation of the problem remains inadequate. While pointing to an important role for institutional discrimination, liberals nonetheless tend to explain racist practices by personal defects of the minority group [60]. In this way the 'culture of poverty' is said to account for differentials in occupation by limiting training, education and work skills. In trying to explain why "Negro voters are weakly organised", Myrdal asserts, "at bottom is the ease with which the Negro masses can be duped - because they are distressed, poorly educated, politically inexperienced, tractable, and have old traditions of dependence and carelessness" [61]. 'Merely giving the solemn promise of equality and liberty' it is argued is not enough to bind intelligent people to American society, since actions speak louder than words!

Ultimately an explanation of the social forces producing racism, or any other fundamental social phenemenon, must take into account economic factors. Only recently have economists investigated the 'problem' of racial discrimination in the labour market. Conservative economists, like Friedman, tend to dismiss the issue: "The maintenance of the general rules of private property and of capitalism have been a major source of opportunity for Negroes" [62]. What inequality does exist reflects personal choice operating within a free labour market:

> It is hard to see that discrimination can have any meaning other than a 'taste' of others that one doesn't share . . . Is there any difference in principle between the taste that leads a householder to prefer an attractive servant to an ugly one and the taste that leads another to prefer a white to a Negro . . . [63]

Other economists have argued that lower wages for blacks reflect economic loss taken by employers who must hire them. Lower productivity, which results from cultural inferiority, and dislike by both the employers and white co-workers for close contact with blacks is said to make it less desirable to hire blacks [64]. The conventional economic approach argues that racism is counter-productive in the economic sphere. Thus employers lose profits, while white workers may gain by preferential access to better jobs. Conservative economists further argue that the free market will eventually eliminate racial discrimination and that workers would be employed solely on the basis of qualification.

The class view proposes an alternative model [65-70]. A comprehensive formulation on this position was first put forward in the late 1960's by the Progressive Labour Party (PLP), a communist organisation which descended from the US Communist Party. The losses suffered by blacks as a result of economic and political discrimination had long been recognised by Communists. It was the impact of racism on white workers which was not understood. In large part as a result of negative experiences in organising black nationalist struggles in the 1960's, the need for multi-racial unity in the class struggle became apparent to the PLP. A thorough-going re-evaluation of the Marxist principle 'racism is also an attack on the white worker' led to a broader and more detailed understanding of the political nature of race. The economic questions were considered primary, as outlined above. Racial discrimination raises profits through 'super-

34

exploitation'. Blacks are forcibly retained in lower-paying, more dangerous jobs, and are paid less for equal work (Tables 2.1, 2.2 and 2.3). They also absorb the brunt of labour practices which allow the employer to lay off workers during a slow period, and also serve as a threat to employed workers who consider changing jobs or striking. But racism is a class weapon; it is equally an attack on white workers. This analysis of racism led to a sharp break with much of the old communist movement, and all nationalist and liberal tendencies. It was to put this programme into practice that the International Committee Against Racism was organised in 1973.

Recent work by Reich and others provides an important test of this theory. Reich bases his analysis on economic data from 48 metropolitan areas in the US in 1960 and 1970. A measure of inequality, the ratio of black to white median income, is taken as an estimate of racism. After adjustment for a number of social factors (region, educational level, per cent employment in industry, etc), Reich demonstrates that as black income goes down 10 per cent, white income at the median falls by 1 per cent. Likewise, the existence of racial differentials is not dysfunctional for the system, rather it boosts profits:

> As increase in racial inequality is associated with a substantial improvement in the share of the richest 1 per cent of white families, with a lesser increase in white inequality overall and with smaller decreases in the share of middle- and lower-income whites. On the basis of these findings, it appears that the redistribution effect of racial inequality is concentrated among the very rich; they are the primary beneficiaries. [71]

An additional important finding of this study, substantiated by several other economists, is the persistence over time of racial differences in income. The median income of black families in 1978 remained at only 57 per cent of that of white families. That is, the median income of blacks was at approximately the same relative level as in the early 1950s [72] (Table 2.4). A modest improvement in relative income occurred over the 1960s; beginning at .54 in 1964 the ratio, black/white, rose to a peak of .61 in 1969, and fell to .57 by

Table 2.1:   Mean Income by Year of School Completed
Males, 25 Years or Older, 1971

Years of School	White	Black	Per Cent Black of White
Less than 8	$ 4984	$ 3912	78
8	6378	4877	76
9-11	8277	5909	71
12	9772	6748	69
13-15	11248	7483	67
16 or more	15355	10684	70

Source: Social Indicators of Equality for
Minorities and Women, US. Commission on Civil Rights

Table 2.2:   Occupation of Male Workers, White and
Nonwhite, 1956

Occupation	Percentage White	Distri-bution Nonwhite	Median Income of occupation
Professional, Technical, Managerial	27	9	$ 7,603
Clerical and Sales	14	9	5,532
Craftsmen and Foremen	20	12	6,270
Operatives	20	27	5,046
Service Workers	6	16	3,436
Non-farm Labourers	6	20	2,410
Farmers and Farm Workers	7	8	1,699

Source: Social and Economic Status of the Black
Population in the US, US Department of Commerce

Table 2.3: Mean Income by Race and Adjustment for
Selected Socio-Economic Variables, Males, 1971 [a]

Race	Raw Values Mean	Ratio to White	Adjusted Values Mean	Ratio to White
Black	$ 7470	.65	$ 9741	.85
Mexican American	7456	.65	9414	.82
Puerto Rican	8269	.72	11233	.98
American Indian	8302	.73	10575	.92
White	11427	1.00	– –	– –

[a] In the case of income, for example, if one
controls for occupational prestige and
education, hours worked last week, and the
average income of the state of residence, black
income increases relative to white but does not
reach it. In 1971 the median raw income among
employed black men was $7470, compared to
$11,427 for white men. When adjusted for the
specific class-related variables listed above
the gap was closed by about half, rising from
65% of that for whites of 85%. An additional
15% is therefore 'unexplained' by the factors
considered and must be ascribed to some other,
independent feature of the race difference. If
blacks and whites were suddenly equal in class
standing blacks would receive 15% lower wages by
virtue of being dark skinned.

Source: Social Indicators or Equality for
Minorities and Women US Commission on Civil Rights.

Table 2.4: Ratio of Nonwhite to White Median Income
United States, 1945-1977

Year	Nonwhite Families	Black Families	Nonwhite Males	Nonwhite Female
1945	.56		n.a.	n.a.
1946	.59		.61	n.a.
1947	.51		.54	n.a.
1948	.53		.54	.49
1949	.51		.49	.51
1950	.54		.54	.49
1951	.53		.55	.46
1952	.57		.55	n.a.
1953	.56		.55	.59
1954	.56		.50	.55
1955	.55		.53	.54
1956	.53		.52	.58
1957	.54		.53	.58
1958	.51		.50	.59
1959	.52		.47	.62
1960	.55		.53	.70
1961	.53		.52	.67
1962	.53		.49	.67
1963	.53		.52	.67
1964	.56	.54	.57	.70
1965	.55	.54	.54	.73
1966	.60	.58	.55	.76
1967	.62	.59	.59	.78
1968	.63	.60	.61	.79
1969	.63	.61	.59	.85
1970	.64	.61	.60	.92
1971	.63	.60	.61	.90
1972	.62	.59	.62	.95
1973	.60	.58	.63	.93
1974	.64	.60	.63	.92
1975	.65	.61	.63	.92
1976	.63	.59	.63	.95
1977	.61	.57	.61	.88

Source: Reich, M. (1981) Racial Inequality: A
Political-economic Analysis, Princeton University
Press, Princeton NJ, pp. 32

Reproduced by kind permission of Princeton
University Press

1977 [73]. These data provide striking confirmation
of the class view of racism and provide a basis for
expanding the analysis of racial discrimination into
other fields, including health.

The history of the race concept - both
scientific and social - has been determined by the
functional role of racism in the capitalist economy.
Racism is not a 'mistake', or a 'failure' of this
society -it is one of its great successes. Race
serves to order human populations and is a perfectly
'natural' concept within the framework of bourgeois
ideology. Liberal critics do not give credit to the
economic origins of racism and concentrate their
attack on its biologic aspects. In effect,
bourgeois science has added nothing fundamental to
an understanding of race since Buffon in 1749. The
concept of race which exists in the popular mind
does not exist on a biological basis; yet race very
much does exist in the social sphere. Thus one
should recognise its existence, and seek to change
the social system that has created it.

By the same token, racism has not been
disappearing. As capitalist society becomes more
powerful, racism becomes more destructive. The last
half century witnessed the most vicious racism
mankind has ever known. Through the Nazi movement
the German ruling class raised race 'science' to new
height, and was able to push it closer to its
logical and necessary conclusion - genocide.
Wage differentials in countries like the US have not
narrowed and the problems of starvation and economic
devastation in the neo-colonial countries grow
larger every day. The North-South economic gulf is
simply a liberal restatement of the racist structure
of imperialism. Maintenance of the status quo in
South Africa appears to have been permanently
accepted by all liberal democracies. In scientific
fields, Burt, Jensen, Wilson and their followers
continue to command great respect and prominence.

The recent historical development of racism
has nonetheless been uneven. On the one hand,
there is greater consciousness about the problems of
race, in large part because of the experience of
fascism and the successes of the anti-racist
movement. On the other hand, the current world-
wide economic downturn has led to the re-emergence
of all the old racist movements, demonstrating the
wellspring of racism in the economic order. Neo-
nazis are prominent in Europe, while the Klu Klux
Klan is given more credibility in the US. More to
the point, the ruling classes of all the major

imperialist countries are becoming more belligerent abroad while intensifying racial divisions at home. The US, Great Britain, Germany, and France have all initiated new anti-immigration campaigns. In recent years Great Britain relived its imperial fantasies in the South Atlantic, the US created the setting for genocide against Palestinian refugees in Lebanon, and the Soviet Union occupied Afghanistan directly and Kampuchea by proxy. The threat of fascism with its racist core of theory and practice threatens our future as it did our parents' future in 1935. Racism is alive and prospering.

RACE AND HEALTH: THE US EXPERIENCE

Unequal life chances are perhaps most starkly and undeniably seen in the physical experience of different social groups within a single country. Racial differentials in health are highly visible in the US, and, in this section, some of the main features of that experience will be outlined. A more detailed examination of the social and biological mechanisms which result in differential mortality by race has been published elsewhere [74].
     Since the discussion will be confined solely to race, it should be placed first within the framework of the other key social determinants of health. The great axes on which the human species is divided, in addition to race, include age, sex, nation and class. While age obviously has a biological component of relevance to health, social factors play a major role in determining the relationship between age and health status [75,76]. The enormous temporal and geographic variation in mortality by age is evidence that external factors are still primary [77]. The health disadvantages suffered by the elderly, and poor children as well, result in large measure from being 'socially un-productive'. Gender plays a complex role in health. In agricultural society women have a shorter life expectancy than men, while in industrialised society the opposite is universally true [78]. The changing pattern of the special oppression of women accounts for these trends; in industrialised society it is men who are subjected to more direct exploitation. National status most clearly resembles the effect of race. The two overlap considerably in the political sphere as well. Finally, class operates vertically within a race or nation and establishes the framework for all other classification. Thus, it

might be argued that race assumes its functional
role by providing the basis for assigning members of
the oppressed racial groups to lower class status.
While it is true that <u>interaction</u> (that is, the
effect of race on class standing) may be the major
effect, the two phenomena are also <u>independent</u>. Age,
sex, nation and race cut across class lines in
separate dimensions. A comprehensive analysis of
race should, therefore, take into account the other
major factors. The present effort is more limited;
the overall structure of differential mortality by
race alone will be described and, with the exception
of class, these questions will not be examined in
detail.

The interaction of class and race cannot be
disregarded; indeed, it might be argued that the
preoccupation with health differences by race has
obscured class questions in the US. Vital records
are not even coded by class background, reflecting
the dissociation of race from class in the official
liberal view. A number of studies are available,
however, which permit an examination of the class-
race interaction. A preliminary analysis is also
possible of what has been called the class effect of
racism; that is, the impact of racial differentials
on the white working class majority.

However, none of these summary statistics
provides a comprehensive view of the trends. For
example, while the ratio relative rate is important,
the absolute difference may follow a divergent
pattern. The relative white-black differential is
greater for women than for men, yet the absolute
difference is less. (Both white and black women
have lower age-adjusted death rates than their male
counter-parts.) Which sex stands at the greater
disadvantage? Other statistics might have been
chosen. In 1970 there were 84,532 excess black
deaths over white [79]. Over half a million person
years were lost to blacks by deaths under the age of
one alone [80].

One must also remain aware of problems with the
vital records. Census undercount and age inflation
lead to inaccuracies among blacks, particularly for
the earlier period. As late as the 1950s a sizable
number of black births took place at home; there is
evidence that many neonatal deaths went
unreported [81]. Acknowledging these limitations,
the overall pattern is nonetheless clear. Despite
enormous changes in social conditions and complete
passage through the epidemiological transition over
the course of this century, black-white

differentials for the major health indices have
improved by one quarter at most. Within this
overall stability dramatic shifts in the type and
character of disease occurred. The underlying
social forces producing discrimination persisted.

Black men suffer an excess mortality from all
the major causes of death compared to whites, with
the exception of suicide (Table 2.5). The largest
absolute excess is found in cancer, with by far the
greatest relative increase in homicide. For
females the same overall pattern applies, with a
more evenly distributed excess (Table 2.5). The
greatest difference in absolute rates is again for
cancer, while homicide show the largest black/white
ratio. Examining the mortality structure, (the
relative importance of each cause of death) allows
the difference in overall death rates to be taken
into account. For black men heart disease is
relatively less important than for whites
(remembering the absolute rates are 10 per cent
higher), and several minor causes contribute a
larger share of deaths (Table 2.6). The mortality
structure for black and white women is more
comparable; specifically, heart disease retains its
relative importance for black women, while cancer is
more important among whites.

Examination of specific causes of death in more
detail confirms the observation that the black
disadvantage is almost universal. Coronary artery
disease (CAD) is by far the most common single cause
of death for both racial groups. Based on the
vital statistics black and white have virtually the
same rates at the present time while death rates for
black women exceed those for white (Table 2.6).
Among middle-aged men, however, blacks are
substantially worse off (Table 2.7). For example
for men ages 55-59 blacks had a CAD death rate of
620 per 100,00 in 1978 while the corresponding
figure for whites was 536. It is the excess of
white deaths in the oldest age groups, or viewed
another way, the deficit of black deaths, that
accounts for the comparable age-adjusted rates.

Is there a different biological pattern to CAD
in blacks than whites? Prospective data are
available from one population-based study and two
large clinical trials [82-84]. Where comparable
groups were studied the risk co-efficients appear to
be similar [85]. Potentially important difference
have been noted in lipoproteins, but this requires
further study. Hypertension clearly plays a
different role in the two groups? Is it possible,

Table 2.5: Death Rates from Major Causes, by Race
and Sex, United States, 1978
(per 100,000 age-adjusted)

Cause of Death	Men White	Men Black	Ratio, B:W	Women White	Women Black	Ratio, B:W
Heart Disease	288.7'	321.0	1.11	136.4	201.1	1.47
Cancer	161.2'	223.7	1.39	109.0	129.2	1.19
Stroke	46.8'	83.8	1.79	39.3	68.7	1.75
Accidents	64.5'	84.0	1.30	22.9	26.1	1.14
Pneumonia	19.6'	33.4	1.70	10.9	15.5	1.42
Suicide	19.2'	12.1	0.63	6.6	3.0	0.45
Cirrhosis	16.1'	30.4	1.89	7.2	14.7	2.04
Diabetes	9.8'	17.4	1.78	9.1	22.4	2.46
Homicide	9.2'	65.6	7.13	2.1	13.5	4.66
Total	773.1'	1113.1	1.44	425.5	650.5	1.53

Source: National Center for Health Statistics
(1981) Health, United States, DHSS Pub. No. (PHS)
82-1232. Public Health Service, Washington DC.

Table 2.6: Contribution to Overall Mortality by
Major Causes, by Race and Sex, United States, 1978

| | % Contribution of Total Mortality | | | |
Cause of Death	Men White	Men Black	Women White	Women Black
Heart Disease	37.3	28.8	32.1	30.9
Cancer	20.9	20.0	25.6	19.9
Stroke	6.1	7.5	9.2	10.6
Accidents	8.3	7.5	5.4	4.0
Pneumonia	2.5	3.0	2.6	2.4
Suicide	2.5	1.1	1.6	0.0
Cirrhosis	2.1	2.7	1.7	2.3
Diabetes	1.3	1.6	2.1	3.4
Homicide	1.2	5.9	0.7	2.1

Source: National Center for Health Statistics (1981)
Health, United States, DHSS Pub. No. (PHS) 82-1232
Public Health Service, Washington DC.

Table 2.7:   Age-Specific Death Rates from CHD
Ages 45-84 1976

Sex and Race	45-54	55-64	65-74	75-84
White Male	275.9	752.2	1697.8	3869.3
Nonwhite Male	326.0	794.5	1487.9	2823.9
White Female	11.7	58.5	730.7	2485.3
Nonwhite Female	148.2	421.8	983.0	2277.8

Source: National   Center   for   Health   Statistics
(1978) Health, United States DHSS Pub. No. (PHS)
78-1232   Public   Health   Service,   Washington DC.

for   example,   that the excess of hypertension leads
to   more   CAD   at a younger age and stroke among the
older   age   groups?   The relative deficit of CAD in
the   oldest   ages   could represent selection.   Death
rates   from all causes are lower among older blacks,
suggesting that some 'health survivor' effect may be
operating [86]. Recent autopsy data from New Orleans
on   persons   in   their   30s   and   40s   who died
accidentally suggest that the prevalence of coronary
atherosclerosis   is   in fact very similar in the two
races in that age range [87].   A recent symposium on
CAD   in blacks was unable to resolve the question of
which   racial   group   had   higher   death rates among
men [88].   For   women, based on the vital statistics
alone,   it   would   appear   that   blacks   have higher
rates.
     The   importance   of   CAD   for   blacks   has been
generally   ignored [89].   As   the   disease, par
excellence,   of middle and upper class white men, it
has   acquired   the   label of a disease of affluence.
The   migration   from   rural   South   to urban North
transformed the social environment of blacks;   these
trends   are   clearly   reflected   in   CAD.   Since the
1950s   blacks   have   smoked   as   much as whites, and
serum   cholesterol   levels are   nearly   equal [90].
Combined   with excess hypertension, this resulted in
a dramatic surge of coronary deaths.
     Cigarettes   are   now among the harmful products
'dumped'   on   the   minority   population.   Whereas 50
years ago in the rural South pellagra was the result
of   poor nutrition among blacks, an excess of animal
fats   and   high-salt,   high-sugar   foods are now the
problems.   They   have   likewise   been excluded from
preventive campaigns.   As the health risk associated
with   smoking   became   known,   campaigns were

selectively aimed at educated whites. A recent
study demonstrated that although blacks had less
prior knowledge about nutrition and CAD, they
learned more than a comparable group of whites over
the study period and experienced greater falls in
serum cholesterol [91]. In sum, 30 years ago blacks
had lower rates of CAD; now, for both sexes
combined, it is more common. The trends in risk
factors are consistent with this epidemiologic
pattern. Commerical forces, primarily sale of
cigarettes and high-profit food items, balanced off
the population's health consciousness, have
determined the level of coronary risk. A similar
time trend, with higher CAD rates initially in the
higher social classes and subsequent reversal, has
also been noted in England [92]. Clearly genetics
does not play an important role in determining the
racial distribution of CAD, the major cause of death
in the US today. Because of the importance of
cardiovascular diseases as a group, hypertension is
by far the single most important influence on
black/white mortality. Prevalence rates for
hypertension in the US are twice as high for blacks
as whites although there is now some very suggestive
evidence that this gap is narrowing. Hypertension
likewise provides the most important example of
potential genetic differences in disease between the
two races. The problem is by no means simple and a
thorough review is well beyond the scope of this
chapter. Hypertension appears to be rare in rural,
isolated African societies [93]. In the larger
cities of West Africa rates of hypertension appear
to be similar to whites in the US and Europe, that
is, around 10 per cent [94]. Blacks of African
descent living in other parts of the world have
twice the usual prevalence, including, Latin
America, the Caribbean, the US and England [95]. A
clear social class gradient for blood pressure
exists (Table 2.8). In the Hypertension Detection
and Follow-up Program, control for weight and
education eliminated racial differences in blood
pressure between women, but not men [96]. (Black men
are not more obese than white men). Although this
question has not been tested directly in other large
studies, the most recent report of the US national
probability survey demonstrates that the social
class gradient persists in both groups [97].
    Although a variety of genetic factors has been
proposed to explain the black/white blood pressure
phenomenon, none is entirely satisfactory [98-101].

Table 2.8:   Hypertension Rates by Race and
Socio-economic Status 1971-1972

Level of Education	Rate of Hypertension White	Black
Less Than 10 Years School	23.1	43.9
10-11 Years	20.8	34.2
12 Years	17.8	29.9
Some College	16.5	27.1
College Graduate	13.5	27.7

Source: Adapted   fom   Hypertension   Detection and
Follow-up   Program   Co-operative   Group   (1977),
Race,   education   and   prevalence   of   hypertension,
American   Journal   of   Epidemiology,   Vol. 106,
pp. 354.

There   is no clear-cut evidence that dietary factors
play   an important role [102].   The putative genetic
sensitivity   to   excess   sodium intake has yet to be
proven.   The   most   consistent   unifying hypothesis
involves   the concept of stress [103].   While racial
oppression   is clearly a concomitant of hypertension
in all black populations, there is no clear evidence
that   it   is   causative.   Difficulties in measuring
and   studying   stress   have   generally   frustrated
efforts   in   this   area.   If   stress   was the major
factor,   it   is   somewhat   surprising   that other
population groups, such as Latinos in the US, do not
have elevated levels of blood pressure.
      An   attempt   to   use   skin   colour   to separate
genetic   effects   in   the US provides an instructive
lesson   in   the   nature   of   race   and   class interactions [104].   Although   lighter-skinned   blacks in
South Carolina had less hypertension than those with
more skin melanin, they were also of a higher social
class [105].   In effect, no separation between class
and race could be made.
      It   must   be   said   that   the   basis   for   the
black/white difference in blood pressure is unknown.
There   could   be   a   genetic predisposition although
the   absence   of   hypertension   in   isolated African
populations demonstrates that the social environment
is   still   the   causative   ingredient.   At   the same
time,   the   narrowing   of   the   black/white   gap by
controlling   for   social   class and obesity suggests
that   much   of   the   difference   relates   to the most
ordinary   social   factors;   furthermore,   it may well

be that neither education nor income are adequate measures of true social status, and that more of the difference could be 'explained'. It goes without saying, of course, that because of racial bias it is almost universally assumed that the observed difference is based on population genetics.

The markedly higher incidence of strokes among blacks can be related to hypertension [106]. The 'stroke belt' in the US is the south-eastern region; it is of interest that not only are rates highest for blacks they are much higher for white in that region as well [107]. Although this point has never been appropriately studied, it seems quite likely that commonly oppressive social conditions could contribute to this association.

Among the neoplastic diseases, blacks suffer an excess for all major sites except leukaemia and breast cancer (Table 2.9) [108]. By far the largest absolute increase occurs for cancer of the lung; among black men rates of prostatic cancer are higher than anywhere else in the world. As a new disease whose social epidemiology is rapidly evolving, breast cancer, like CAD, is becoming more common among blacks, while declining slightly for whites.

Lung cancer, particularly among men, is the overwhelming source of the differential in death from this category. A number of unusual epidemiological features have been observed. Lung cancer rates among white men began to rise rapidly in the middle third of this century, afflicting the generation born around 1900 who took up smoking in the 1920s and 1930s [109]. Rates for blacks took off about 10 years later, but with a slope that was twice as steep. By the 1950s black men aged 35–54 had already passed their white counterparts and by 1980 rates among the maximally effected cohort of blacks were twice those for the corresponding generation of whites (Table 2.10). Curiously, not until the late 1950s did smoking rates among blacks equal those for whites [110]. Why has the disease been more severe? Certainly blacks now smoke more, but that is an insufficient explanation of the trends over the last 50 years. Some improvement in recording of death certificates could have played a role, but that is also not an adequate explanation by itself.

Two potential factors can be cited: occupation and low pro-vitamin A (carotene) intake. Industrial occupations are an important source of exposure to pulmonary carcinogens, and there is no question but that blacks are more exposed at the work

Race, Disease and Health

Table 2.9:   Cancer Death Rates by Race, United
States, 1976, Age-adjusted (per 100,000)

| | Male | | Female | |
Cause of Death	White	Nonwhite	White	Nonwhite
All Cancer	159.1	202.3	108.2	119.3
Digestive Organ	40.3	57.3	26.3	32.2
Respiratory	55.6	68.2	14.8	14.2
Breast	0.2	0.4	23.3	20.8
Genital Organs	14.1	25.0	14.9	20.7
Other	48.9	51.4	28.9	21.3

Source: National Center for Health Statistics
Vital Statistics of the United States, Vol. II
1976-1977, Public Health Service, DHEW, Hyattsville,
MD.

Table 2.10: Cancer of the Lung, White and Non-
white, United States, 1930-77
Rate per 100,000

Age-Race Group	1930	1940	1950	1960	1970	1977	%Increase 1950-77
White							
45-54	8	20	35	54	68	74	+111
55-64	13	41	85	152	199	209	+146
Non-white							
45-54	3	15	34	72	113	131	+285
55-64	6	20	69	159	232	305	+342

Source: National Center for Health Statistics,
Vital Statistics of the United States, Vol. II,
1930-1977 Public Health Service, DHEW Hyattsville
MD.

place [111,112]. Unfortunately, no national surveys
are available to provide an estimate of the overall
magnitude of this problem. It may be that a
relatively small number of individuals are
sufficiently exposed. Carotene intake has been shown
to be a powerful protective factor against lung
cancer [113]; intake of this micro-nutrient is lower
among blacks reflecting fewer vegetables in the
diet [114]. It is also possible that the
concentration of blacks in urban centres, where air
pollution is worse, could be a factor. At any rate,
the secular trends alone provide irrefutable
evidence that the root cause is again social
conditions. All the leading contenders for
explanation of the mechanism point to the effects of
racial discrimination.

Violence — taking homicide and accidents
collectively — contributes significantly to the
increased mortality among blacks, particularly males
between the ages of 15 and 35 [115]. The social
origins of this cause of death need not be
elaborated. A recent ecological study of homicide
provides a useful exposition of the process of
controlling for social class [116]. Based on the
experience in Atlanta, Georgia, the question was
addressed, do blacks have a specific 'culture of
violence'? That is, for a similar set of social
conditions, are rates higher among blacks than
whites? Controlling for education alone, a
sizable difference remained. However, it was noted
that even with identical education blacks receive
lower wages. Substituting income further narrowed
the gap although it was not closed. Because of
segregation, black purchasing power is also well
below that of whites; similar housing costs up to
30 per cent more in a segregated black
neighbourhood. The racial difference disappeared
altogether when using occupants per room as a direct
measure of purchasing power. Stepwise elimination
of race differences by controlling for class
variables is a virtually universal finding. It
should not be taken to mean, however, that race is
not the cause of the difference.

Death from cirrhosis is twice as common among
blacks as whites, for both sexes. National estimates
of drinking habits generally show equal intake
overall; use of alchohol is likewise positively
associated with income [117]. Despite these
findings it would appear that blacks in the age
range vulnerable for alcoholism (that is 15 to 35),
have a higher rate of this eminently social disease.

The epidemiology of diabetes presents further paradoxes. While death rates are twice as high among blacks, glucose tolerance appears to be somewhat better [118]. The occurrence of diabetes in persons who have other illnesses, such as hypertension, may explain the higher mortality among blacks although this hypothesis was not confirmed in a recent study [119].

A host of more minor causes of death fill out the picture of racial differentials. Blacks have greater rates of end-stage renal disease and lupus erythematosus, and one does simply not know whether or not this results from greater exposure to viral illnesses and other pollutant antigens of the big city. At the other end of the spectrum of 'new versus old diseases' blacks continue to experience higher rates of traditional infectious killers, such as tuberculosis and venereal diseases.

Mechanisms of Differential Mortality

To the extent that specific mechanisms can be identified, differential black/white mortality can be explained by the concept of super-exploitation. Occupational disease is the most straightforward example. In the US, however, job-related illness represents only a small proportion of the total disease burden. At the other end of the production-consumption cycle, cigarettes and poor nutrition are the major killers. Living conditions, in terms of the home environment, popular culture, unemployment and so on, contribute to the epidemics of addiction, homicide, psychiatric disorders and, perhaps, hypertension. The life style of capitalism creates a spectrum of disease across these three inter-related spheres. Lung cancer can be related to occupation and cigarette consumption. CAD is cased by cigarettes and hypertension and a diet high in animal products. Alcoholism reflects, at least in part, the marketing pressures of the liquor industry. These diverse disease-producing forces are focused in excess on the minority population by racism.

The purpose of super-exploitation is to raise the profitability of capitalism. The two principal forms this takes are lowering of wages and providing a more controlled, even monopolistic, consumer market [120]. The relative importance of the producer versus the consumer role in racist super-exploitation varies with historical conditions although the sphere of production remains the

primary source of excess profits. It is estimated,
however, that being confined to a controlled
consumer market, with its gross distortions of true
needs, in combination with hazardous living
conditions, account for the majority of the black
health disadvantage in the US. In South Africa, by
contrast, aside from consumption of cigarettes,
alcohol and the barest necessities of life, blacks
fulfil almost exclusively a productive role.
Without a diet high in animal products, CAD is
virtually absent, and cancer, hypertension, violence
and infection/undernutrition determine the structure
of mortality [121-123]. Consumption, therefore,
plays a minor role.
     In the US black population, the mortality
structure might accurately be viewed as an
intensification of the experience of the industrial
white working class, where all the raw edges have
been sharpened. Not only are total death rates
higher but there is also more wastage of life from
the 'older', violent and more readily preventable
causes. In search for true causative mechanisms,
however, the existence of racial differentials
cannot be 'explained' by social class. Accounting
for education and income for instance, in the
effort to explain racial differentials represents
over-control; that is, race is not confounded by
the other variables, it is antecedent to them. The
health disadvantage of blacks cannot be eliminated,
for example, by better education. Only an explicit,
social campaign to attack the obstacles to more
education (that is, racism) will be effective. An
even more simplistic analytic error is often made:
biological variables, such as obesity, blood
pressure, and others, are used to explain the health
disadvantage of blacks. Clearly these are only
attributes, not causes. Ascribing inferior health
status to exposure to the more dangerous environment
accepts as given precisely the thing to be
explained. Health status can only be understood as
a social phenomenon.

Explaining the Mechanism of Change
The explanation of the difference in health status
between blacks and whites appears straightforward,
from a conceptual point of view. The mechanisms
which determine this structure, however, are more
complicated. Cause-specific analysis is necessary
to elucidate the biological mechanisms which result
in higher death rates for blacks although the

51

general process of racial super-exploitation remains
constant. By the same token, according to Reich's
economic model [124], analysis that predicts the
changes in the intensity of racism would have a
primary effect on black mortality, with an important
secondary effect on the health of the white working
class.

Infant mortality is widely regarded as a key
indicator of the quality of life of a population.
Over the last 40 years the black/white ratio in
infant mortality has been very constant, suggesting
some consistent underlying relationship (figure
2.3). Black disadvantage can in large part be
attributed to poverty although, as in many other
areas, higher mortality is noted even when mothers
have 'comparable' income, education and medical
care [125-127]. The biological factors are best
captured by the variables of prematurity and low
birthweight [128].

The analysis of possible class effects was
based on vital records for infant deaths from 28 US
cities having populations of over 500,000 for the
years 1965 to 1978 [129]. Race-adjusted rates were
used to compare cities, and the ratio of black/white
infant mortality was taken as a measure of racial
inequality of health status. In Table 2.11 a
correlation matrix of the mortality data and several
sociological variables is presented. Both white and
black infant mortality correlate strongly with the
estimate of the racial disparity expressed in the
ratio of death rates in the two groups. The
segregation index was not significantly related to
the mortality levels.

Multiple regression analysis was also performed
with the race-adjusted rate as the dependent
variable (Table 2.12). By far the greatest
predictive value was noted for the racial ratio.
Overall 41 per cent of the variance in the rates was
accounted for by this equation. It would appear
that the parallel downward trend in black and white
infant death rates has been linked to a common trend
in social conditions. The accelerated decline in
the 1960s could well reflect the improvement in the
social status which occurred at that time. However,
that explanation by itself is not sufficient. The
degree of racial disparity, as a reflection of the
intensity of racism, is an additional determinant of
the level of mortality for both groups. Whether
this finding is specific to big cities in this
period remains to be determined. To the extent

Figure 2.3:   Infant Mortality Rates by Race: 1935-1978

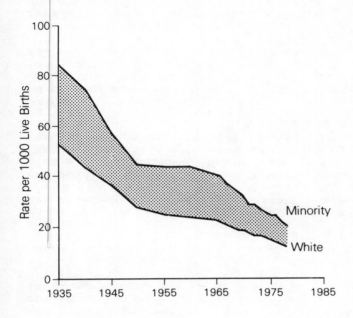

Table 2.11: Race and Infant Mortality in United
States' Cities; Correlation Matrix

	B IMR	B:W Ratio	Pct B'65	Pct B'78	Seg Index	Rac Adj IMR
W IMR[a]	.64	(.09)	.50	.53	(-.01)	.95
B IMR		.82	(.03)	(.18)	(.03)	.82
B:W Ratio			(-.33)	(-.16	(.04)	(.36)
Pct B '65				.86	(-.10)	(.38)
Pct B '78					(-.25)	.43
Seg Index						(-.04)

[a] WIMR = white infant mortality rate
    BIMR = black infant mortality rate
    B:W Ratio = ratio, B IMR:W IMR
    Pct B '65 = percent of population B in 1965
    Pct B '78 = percent of population B in 1978
    Seg Index = index of residential segregation
    Race Adj IMR = race adjusted IMR
    P-values for co-efficients, N=21
       (r)   p
       .43   .05
       .54   .01
       .58   .005
       .65   .001

Source: David, R. and Reis, J. Race and Infant
Mortality in US Cities.   Effects of Race-specific
Mortality Rates and Black/white Differentials,
Unpublished Manuscript, pp. 81

Table 2.12: Race and Infant Mortality in
United States' Cities; Regression Analysis

(N=21) Variable	Sum of Squares	F. Value
Total	.1378	– –
Regression	.0571	2.79
B:W Ratio	.0317	6.20
Pct B '65	.0198	3.87
Pct B '78	.0056	1.09
Seg Index	.0001	02
Residual	.0818	– –

R^2 = 0.4112
[a] See Table 2.13 for variable labels

Source: David, R. and Reis, J. Race and Infant
Mortality in US Cities.   Effects of Race-specific
Mortality Rates and Black/white Differentials,
Unpublished Manuscript, pp. 81

Race, Disease and Health

that they can be generalised, these findings corroborate the outcome of Reich's econometric analysis [130].

A second study was carried out on the mortality experience of the adult population [131]. Marked improvement in health status took place for the black population between 1968 and 1978 (Table 2.13). Life expectancy for black men increased 4.6 years while for black women the increase was 5.7 years. Examining the relative black/white changes over this period, the decline in death rates for all causes for the age group 35-74 was found to be greater for blacks than whites. For men, this represented a 10.5 per cent reduction in the mortality ratio, and for women a 31.1 per cent decrease (Table 2.14). This was the first period since the 1930s that the racial gap had been narrowed. Hypertension detection and control, with the decline in cardio-vascular deaths, appeared to play the major role. Abundant evidence exists to indicate that access to health care became more equally distributed as a result of the mass anti-racist struggles of the 1960s and early 1970s [132,133].

Although temporal association by itself is not proof, it would seem clear enough that the period of progressive change in the US led directly to dramatic improvement in health. Blacks benefited most - in both absolute and relative terms - yet whites shared a considerable proportion of the positive effects. In summarising the health trends over this period, one might say that the racial differential for adults was narrowed by 15-20 per cent. At the same time, the progressive energy released by the anti-racist movement benefited the entire working class. A more detailed analysis using direct estimates of anti-racist change, as performed with infant mortality, might help refine this point; however, the general conclusions are not vulnerable to the strict positivist critique. Much stands to be gained in the short run from organised opposition to racial oppression, by both blacks and whites.

Racism as an International Problem
The problem of race is international, in two senses. First, racial differentials exist all over the world. Almost all modern nations have sub-populations which are subjected to racial discrimination. The variety is almost endless. In

55

Table 2.13: Mortality Rates from All Causes,
Age-Adjusted, Persons Age 35-74, by Sex-Colour
(Rate per 100,000)

Year	White Men	White Women	Non-white Men	Non-white Women
1968	2119.7	1064.9	2919.8	1883.8
1978	1738.2	879.4	2331.8	1345.9
Change:	-381.5	-185.5	-588.0	-537.9
Percent Change:	-18.0%	-17.4%	-20.1%	- 28.6%

Source: National Center for Helath Statistics
Vital Statistics of the United States, Vol. II
1968, 1978 Public Health Service, Washington DC.

Table 2.14: Ratio of Death Rates, Non-white:
White, 1968 and 1978 Selected Causes, Persons
Age 35-74, by Sex

| Mortality Cause | SEX-COLOUR GROUP AND YEAR | | | |
| | Men | | Women | |
	1968	1978	1968	1978
Coronary Heart Disease	0.99	0.98	1.66	1.51
Stroke	2.19	2.09	2.64	2.16
Non-Cardiovascular	1.53	1.50	1.57	1.38
All Causes	1.38	1.34	1.77	1.53

Source: National Center for Health Statistics,
Vital Statistics of the United States, Vol. II,
1968,1978 Public Health Service, Washington DC.

India and Japan remnants of the caste system persist. Aboriginal populations in Australia, Canada, New Zealand and the US suffer permanent social disadvantage. Majority ethnic groups in Bolivia and South Africa are enslaved by the colonial descendants. Soviet minority republics experience unequal living conditions although their position improved enormously in the first part of this century. Guest workers in Europe, Israel, Africa and the US all face sharp restrictions of economic and political opportunity. Within each form of racial oppression economic advantage results for those in power, and poor health for the exploited.

The second aspect of the international problem of race reflects the imperialist division of the world into what are commonly called 'developed' and 'under-developed' countries. This structure has also been referred to as the 'three worlds'. In fact, neither of those concepts is satisfactory. Poor countries are neither 'under-developed' nor in a separate world. They have a fully developed relationship with the world economy, namely that of a neo-colony. A more appropriate theoretical construct is that of a unitary three-tiered structure, composed of central or dominant countries (US, USSR, Japan, and their closest allies), peripheral industrialised countries (such as southern Europe), and neo-colonies (most of Africa, Latin America, and Asia). Within the imperialistic world economy a health pattern can be described which reflects this political structure and has determinants beyond measures of average wealth.

Although detailed analysis of this question is beyond the scope of this chapter, the essential features can be summarised as follows. The experiences of the central industrial countries has been described in preceding sections. Atherosclerosis, cancer, addiction and violence are the primary disease forces. The period of rapid economic development has been associated with an upturn in adult mortality of men; in some countries these trends have been sufficient to result in sizable reduction in life expectancy [134–138]. Consumptive factors play the major role in the production of these epidemics [139]. The peripheral countries generally do not experience the new epidemic with equal force although they enjoy similar marked declines in infant death rates; as a result life expectancy may be longer or similar at

lower levels of per capita Gross National Product
(GNP). Italy, for example, enjoys a longer life
expectancy than the US, with only one quarter the
per capita wealth [140].

The mortality structure of the neo-colonial
countries is likewise historically unique [141-144].
It does not represent an earlier stage of the same
path of development which the central countries
experienced. The primary feature of this health
disadvantage relates to undernutrition and
infection, particularly among the young. Based on
a data set comprised of mortality statistics from 43
countries over the last century, Preston
demonstrates the unique features of this
pattern [145]. In Table 2.15, neo-colonial
countries are matched with European countries or the
US during the period in which levels of total
mortality were comparable. As noted by Preston,
"In every non-Western population, diarrheal death
rates either equal or exceed the average rates among
the Western populations used as a standard" [146].
Tuberculosis, while common in the neo-colonies, does
not reach the level recorded for the urban working
class of early industrialisation. These findings
have been substantiated in a recent detailed study
of Latin America [147]. A comparison of mortality
in the US and Latin America demonstrates that the
industrialised countries (for example the US and
Argentina) enjoy most of their advantage in infancy
(Table 2.16). In fact rising infant death rates
are now a feature of several neo-colonies [148-150].

The relationship between per capita wealth and
mortality is not linear across the three tiers of
imperialist countries. First, at a certain level
the relationship flattens [151]. That is, when the
new epidemics reach sufficient strength, no more net
decline in adult death rates takes place. Second,
in the neo-colonies, particularly in the last two
decades, rising per capita income has only had a
very small effect on mortality [152]. This
disruption of the historical relationship between
rising average wealth and falling death rates
probably reflects the higher degree of inequality in
distribution of wealth which exists in those
countries [153-155]. In effect, large segments of
the population, primarily peasants driven from the
land, become of marginal value in the 'human
capital' equation, and are literally thrown out to
starve.

A further reflection of this process has been
the pattern of increase in life expectancy. In the

Table 2.15: Comparison of Death Rates from Respiratory
Tuberculosis, Other Infections and Parasitic Diseases,
and Diarrhea in Non-western Populations in the 1960s
With those in Western Populations at Equivalent
Mortality Levels (per 100,000)

| | | AGE ADJUSTED DEATH RATE FROM SPECIFIED CAUSE | | |
Population Group and Year	All Causes	Respiratory Tuberculosis	Other Infections and Parasitic	Diarrhea
Non-Western				
Ceylon, 1960	1155	15	48	49
Chile, 1964	1196	37	43	44
Columbia, 1964	1188	26	71	66
Guatemala, 1964	1840	36	305	231
Mexico, 1964	1152	23	63	85
South Africa (coloured) 1960	1666	85	64	194
Western				
France, 1926	1625	115	53	47
England and Wales, 1901	1971	106	169	107
Ireland, 1951	1211	54	26	8
Sweden, 1930	1159	105	61	15
United States 1970	1159	33	28	12

Source: Adapted from Preston, S.H. (1976) Mortality Patterns in
National Populations, Academic Press, New York, pp. 40.

Table 2.16: A Comparison of Infant and Adult
Mortality in the United States and Selected
Latin American Countries, 1965

	Country	Infant Mortality (per 1,000)	All Causes, Ages 55-64 (per 100,000)
I	Latin America		
	Columbia	82.4'	17.6
	Venezuela	75.3'	18.5
	Guatemala	92.6	16.4'
	Argentina	56.9	18.3
	Peru	74.0	18.2
	Mexico	60.7'	17.1
	Chile	95.4	13.8
	Mean	76.8	17.1
II	United States	24.7'	16.4

Source: United Nations, Demographic Yearbooks, 1966,
1967, United Nations, New York.

first two decades after World War II, life expectancy in the neo-colonies rose more rapidly than at comparable periods for the central countries. This phenomenon was attributed primarily to the export of technological progress, in health as well as other fields [156]. It is now apparent that the trajectory of lengthening life expectancy has changed. Stagnation is taking place in the neo-colonies at an absolute level well below that of the central and peripheral industrialised countries [157]. The current world-wide economic downturn falls most cruelly on the heavily-indebted neo-colonies. Future trends are likely to demonstrate a worsening of this health pattern.

The imperialist division of the world has many inter-related structural supports, not the least of which is military force. Nonetheless, racism plays a major role in justifying the political and economic dominance of the central imperialist powers. The unique public health characteristics noted above - predominance of diarrheal disease, disruption of the relationship between per capita income and mortality, and the truncation of the life expectancy curve - reflect the special features of racism in the international perspective. Just as with the health disadvantage of blacks in the US, the neo-colonies suffer permanent restriction within the current world-wide economic system. Extraction of wealth, in terms of raw materials, agriculture products, and cheap labour, is the equivalent form taken by super-exploitation.

RACISM AND HEALTH CARE SERVICES IN THE US

Racial segregation is deeply rooted in the US medical care system. The first hospitals for blacks, such as Lincoln in New York City, Freedmen's in Washington, DC, and Provident in Chicago, were established in the 19th century to care for blacks who escaped from the South; all three function today as almost exclusively minority institutions. As part of the 'Flexnerian Revolution' in the first decades of this century, two black medical schools, Meharry and Howard, were endowed by the Rockefeller Foundation and other philanthropies to produce black doctors who could serve as the basis for a separate health care system. Through the 1940s some state branches of the AMA excluded blacks and most hospitals in the South did not accept them on their staff. Until the 1980s most private hospitals in the South did not even admit black patients, and if they did so it was onto strictly segregated wards. Until the late 1960s, state laws prohibited cross-racial transfusions.

Civil rights legislation of the 1960s and federal medical payment plans such as Medicaid had a significant impact on segregation in health care, particularly in the South. The US however still operates a two-class health system divided by race. A recent study confirmed that in a large, multi-racial northern city like New York a 'separate and unequal' health care system remains intact. Twenty-four of the total 94 hospitals studied had an in-patient census which was less than 10 per cent non-white [158]. At the other extreme 7 hospitals were more than 80 per cent non-white. The proportion of patients covered by Medicaid was strongly related to race in multiple regression analysis. Based on two quality-of-care indicators, namely nurse-to-patient ratio and total assets, hospitals with more non-white patients ranked lower. Within-hospital segregation was not accounted for in this study and would most likely widen the racial inequality.

Measuring overall rates of utilisation, racial differentials for the country as a whole have narrowed considerably over the last decade and a half [159]. Even taking into account greater need among blacks, their disadvantage is relatively slight [160]. However, quality of care is not easily measured. Two useful indicators of quality of care include hypertension detection and control and cancer survival rates. Blacks are now only slightly less likely to have their hypertension controlled than are whites [161]. This remarkable development no doubt reflects the expansion of services in the 1970s, and as was noted earlier it may have played a crucial role in reducing the black/white mortality differential among adults. On the other hand, controlling for stage of diagnosis blacks have lower five year survival rates for all major tumors [162]. This is especially marked for the more treatable tumors, for example colon (black = 35 per cent, white = 46) compared to lung (black = 6, white = 9) [163].

Racism and Reaction: Current Trends
Unfortunately, the crucial role of anti-racism in the social transformations of the 1960s and 1970s is more than matched by the role of racism in ushering in the present era of reaction. Driven by the

recession and rising international tensions, the
ruling elite has been forced to rely on an
intensification of racism in their efforts to
prevent the social system from unravelling.
Medical care is playing a crucial role in the
development and the main features of this process
are outlined here.

Leibel, writing in the New England Journal as
early as 1976, noted that over the previous two
years there had been a major shift in perspective in
the medical literature from enthusiasm to
demoralisation and scepticism [164]. The concept of
'shrinking resources' was being translated into
strategies to limit and ration health services. The
'Living Will' was developed and a new national
debate on euthanasia emerged [165-168]. Cost-benefit
analysis was proposed as the fundamental tool for
medical and public health decision-making. Instead
of cost versus benefit for the individual patient,
the issue was now what 'society' had to gain. For
example, it has been argued that screening for lead
poisoning is not cost efficient if the prevalence
is less than 6 per cent; long term
institutionalisation of retarded children is
cheaper [169]. While these 'theoretical' discussions
are carried out screeening programmes are
eliminated. It is, of course, apparent that with a
prevalence of 12 per cent among black children and 2
per cent among white, the abolition of screening
programmes for lead poisoning exacts a different
price in health from the two groups [170]; a price,
nonetheless, paid by both. Racism has likewise been
important in the process of closing hospitals. The
New York City segregation study demonstrated that
the in-patient racial composition was an important
independent predictor of hospital closure [171]. The
attack on health care for the elderly represents a
parallel development. Some authors argue, in total
contradiction of the facts, that "the medical and
social task of eliminating premature death is
largely accomplished" [172]. Others propose that
the time has come to "allow persons who are demented
or likely to die within a few months to die without
the intervention of modern medicine" [173]. In fact,
it is clear that the potential of longevity has by
no means been exhausted [174]. By the same token,
the present day euthanasia movement bears an
unmistakable resemblance to its predecessors [175];

saving capital is its reason for existence. While preventive measures and 'death with dignity' are posed as hypothetical alternatives they never take a practical form.

What is the strategy of those who seek to reduce health services? Doctors much prefer to offer treatment, and particularly in the US are reimbursed in like measure. Undermining the activist character of contemporary medicine requires an agressive campaign. While all the traditional forms of reactionary ideology have been called into play, racism has the key role. At a 'Private Sector Conference' Daniel Tosteson, Dean of Harvard Medical School, sounded the call for a retreat from the promise of equality in health care [176]. Arguing that "societal pressures were demanding a reduction in the unit cost of each health service", Tosteson asked rhetorically; "Doesn't this mean a return to a multi-class system"? First on the list for cuts has been Medicaid. As Rogers et al, point out, the racism is clear: "Medicaid has become identified in the minds of the public as simply another form of welfare payment to a narrow group of unemployed adults and minorities" [177]. Rogers et al, further acknowledged that the attack on Medicaid gravely threatens the white working class:

> in reality, it (Medicaid) provides care to a broad cross-section of people in the United States. It includes primarily elderly people who are retired, people who are blind or who are severely disabled over a longer term, poor children, and only a very few adults who are temporarily unemployed. Likewise . . . less than 30 per cent of the program's funds support services for minorities. [178]

Federal health programmes have been severely cut in the US. These reductions, however, are nowhere near large enough to meet the demands of the growing military build up. Further reductions must include the private sector. Now that an ideological justification for reductions has been established, a broader scope of operation can be undertaken. It would appear that the AMA as the single most powerful medical organisation and the representative of private physicians has been given this task. Rationing life has become the new cause of the AMA [179,180]. In a recent series of articles this

position was outlined in some detail; a summary
editorial appears in Figure 2.4.

At the conclusion of a detailed argument in
support of rationing based on social utility, Evans
makes this comment:

> analogies are likely to be made between
> current events and the events that took place
> in Nazi Germany . . . The practice of rationing
> will bring forth cries that the precedent is
> now set for the floodgates to be opened to the
> 'mass slaughter' of persons whom rationing
> criteria declare to be of 'marginal value'
> [181].

There is good reason to believe that this is
entirely correct, yet what response does Evans
offer? "The point of the matter is that rationing
decisions are already being made" (which eliminate
persons of marginal value).

Eliminating those of marginal value, who are
'primarily consumptive rather than productive' is,
of course, the basic strategy of Nazi medicine. An
extensive literature exists on the fascist
transformation of medicine in the 1920s and 1930s,
and it was not confined to Germany alone [182-185].
Beginning with the publication of "The Destruction
of Life Devoid of Value" in 1920 by Binding and
Hoche, a growing movement within medicine demanded
the elimination of 'people of marginal value'. The
criteria proposed by the AMA (Figure 2.4) fit like a
glove the Nazi definition of 'useless eaters'.
During the years around 1940, 275,000 mental
patients were exterminated, as were many thousands
of 'handicapped' children as well [186]. It is
important to recognise that these campaigns were
proposed, organised and carried out primarily by
doctors acting without direct orders of the Nazi
party [187]. They were simply putting into practice
an ideology which they had come fully to accept.
It goes without saying that racism was the heart and
soul of that ideology. Once it became accepted that
some human beings were inferior and no longer
deserved to live, the aggressive forces of class
society were unleashed in unspeakably vicious ways.
Only the ideology of racism could have made that
development possible.

Similar historical conditions exist on many
levels today. From unemployment to the level of
military tension, analogies to the 1930s abound.

Figure 2.4   Rationing Human Life

"Its not the length of a man's life that matters,
it's the quality." Martin Luther King

What is a human life worth? Is each human life
worth the same as every other? Or does the worth of
a human life depend on the following:
   * What country, state, county, or city a person
lives in?
   * The color of a person's skin, the language
spoken, the person's age, gender, or sexual
preference?
   * Whether the person:
     Has an IQ of 150 or less than 50?
     Is a heart surgeon or a jaundiced nexborn?
     Is a concert violinist or a victim of trisomy
        21?
     Is a star professional quarterback or a
        quadriplegic?
     Is a millionaire or is on welfare?
     Is a mother of five young children or is a
        convicted rapist?
     Is a practicing psychologist or an
        institutionalized schizophrenic?
     Is a social worker or an active street heroin
        addict?
     Is a celebrated ethicist or a functional
        illiterate?
     Is primarily productive or primarily
        consumptive?
These questions are being asked and choices are now
made on a daily case-by-case basis. We all know
that in virtually all societies, rank has its
privileges. Is life itself one of these
privileges?

Source: Editorials, Journal of the American Medical
Association, vol. 249, No. 16, pp. 2223

Reproduced by kind permission of the American
Medical Association

While profound differences do also exist, these periods are two identical cycles in the historical process of the decay of the capitalist world system. Dealing as it does with life and death issues on a daily basis, medicine will always play a key role in ushering in a new era of fascism.

Before leaving this section, the broader implications of these questions must be reinforced. It is by no means to be understood that elimination of medical services for a disproportionate segment of the minority population will be the only consequence of current developments in medicine. Society exists as an organic whole, with all its parts highly inter-related. The economic forces at work today, while they may be temporarily abated, are leading to eventual collapse of the current financial system. The ruling elite will be forced to resort to fascism to meet these new conditions. At the same time, for both internal and external reasons, the two great imperialist powers may well be driven into conflict. These events are in general terms a reproduction of the period from 1930 to 1945. The level of destruction of human life which will result from World War III far exceeds the losses which will result from intensified domestic racism. If roughly 4 million died in WWI, and 40 million in WWII, then the Pentagon estimate of 400 million in WWIII falls along the appropriate regression line. Racism has a dynamic quality, releasing tremendous energy from within the ordinary constraints of class society; the output tends to exceed equivalent input. This chain reaction can serve the cause of anti-racism, and multiply the advantage for the non-white majority, or it can be marshalled to serve the purposes of fascism and lead to slaughter beyond comprehension. The importance of anti-racism, even in relation to health, cannot be understood within the narrow context of differential mortality. Just as it grows out of fundamental structural contradictions of the capitalist system, its growth or dissipation affects all of society in profound ways.

CONCLUSIONS

In the sense that man's basic social impulse is to master history, it is not the human view of the world to look on the savagery of racism and turn one's back and walk away. Health is our window on the world; through it we see the vitality and

infinite pleasure of living strangled by 'a hideous
god who will drink only from the skulls of murdered
men'. Let us remember that Wounded Knee, Treblinka,
Babi Yar, Soweto, Attica, Asam, Mai Lai, Derry, and
al Sabra/Shatilla did not fall from the sky. They
are the creations of our social system. They were
perpetuated by the masters of this world in their
pursuit of progress. Yet with ever-greater urgency
the question is forced upon us. Is this the only
path human progress can take?

Only an organised social movement can intervene
against this epidemic. Unfortunately, the anti-
racist movement today is far too small; it cannot
meet the enemy with anything approaching equal
force. Yet the long-term advantage is on our side.
The reserve army for the cause of anti-racism can
be counted in the billions. On the threat of
extermination the world's people will be driven to
answer in practice the questions raised here.
Health workers concerned not about careers and
salaries and job security but health in its
broadest, most fundamental sense should seek to lead
this movement.

REFERENCES

1. Montague, A. (ed) (1964) The Concept of Race,
      Collier-Macmillan, Toronto
2. Dobzhansky, T. (1973) Genetic Diversity and
      Human Equality, Basic Books, New York
3. Boyd, W.C. (1963) Genetics and the Human Race,
      Science Vol. 140, pp. 1057-1064
4. Woodward, V. (1981) Heredity and Human Society,
      Burgess Publishing Company, Minneapolis
5. Chase, A. (1980) The Legacy of Malthus: The
      Social Costs of the New Scientific Racism,
      University of Illinois Press, Champaign,
      IL
6. Gossett, T.F. (1965) Race: the History of an
      Idea in America, Shocken Books, New York
7. Referred to in Montague, A. (1964) op. cit. pp.
      3
8. Watt, E.S. (1981) The biological race concept
      and the diseases of modern man, in H.R.
      Rothschild, (ed) Biocultural Aspects of
      Disease, Academic Press, New York, pp. 3-
      22

9. Ehrlich, P.R., Holm R.W. (1964) A biological
    view of race, in A. Montague (ed.) The
    Concept of Race, Collier-Macmillan,
    Toronto, pp. 153-197
10. Boyd, W.C.(1950) Genetics and the Races of
    Man, Little Brown and Company, Boston, pp.
    186-209
11. Watt, E.S. (1981) op. cit., pp. 11
12. Montague, A. (1964) op. cit.
13. Gould, S.J. (1979) Ever Since Darwin:
    Reflections in Natural History, W.W.
    Norton Company, New York
14. Dobzhansky, T (1962) Comment of Livinstone,
    Current Anthropology, Vol. 3, pp. 279-280
15. Dobzhansky, T., Ayala F.J., Stebbins, and G.L.,
    Valentine J.W., (1977) Evolution, W.H.
    Freeman, San Francisco
16. Coon, C.S. (1962) The Origin of Races, Knopf,
    New York
17. Barnicot, N.A. (1954) Taxonomy and variation in
    modern man, in A. Montague (ed) The
    Concept of Race, Collier-Macmillan,
    Toronto, pp. 180-227
18. Dobzhansky, et al (1977) op. cit.
19. Watt, E.S. (1981) op. cit., pp. 11
20. Coon, C.S. (1962) op. cit.
21. Montague, A. (1964) op. cit.
22. Boyd, W.C. (1950) op. cit.
23. Montague, A. (1964) op. cit., pp. 177
24. Watt, E.S (1981) op. cit.
25. Dobzhansky T. (1982) op. cit.
26. Dobzhansky, T. et al, (1977) op. cit.
27. Coon, C.S. (1962) op. cit.
28. Dobzhansky, T. (1962) op. cit., pp. 280
29. Dobzhansky, T. et al (1977) op. cit.
30. Ibid., pp. 163
31. Ibid., pp. 145
32. Ibid., pp. 145
33. Glass, B. (1943) Genes and the Man, Columbia
    University Press, New York
34. Boyd, W.C. (1950) op. cit.
35. Lewontin, R.C.(1972) Apportionment of human
    diversity, Evolutionary Biology, Vol. 6,
    pp. 381-398
36. Dobzansky, T. et al (1977) op. cit.

37. Dunn, F.G., Oigman, W., Sungaard-Rise, K., Messerli, F.H., Ventura, H., Reisin, and . E. Frohlic, (ed) (1983) Racial differences in cardiac adaptation to essential hypertension determined by echocardio-graphic indexes, Journal of the American College of Cardiology Vol. 1, pp. 1348-51

38. Paul, J.R. (1957) The Epidemiology of Rheumatic Fever, American Heart Association, New York

39. Newsholme, A. (1895) Milroy Lectures: rheumatic fever, Lancet Vol. 1, pp. 589-596, 657-665

40. Stollerman, G H (1975) Rheumatic Fever and Stretococcal Infection, Grune and Stratton, New York

41. Ibid.

42. Montague, A. (1964) op. cit. pp. xii

43. Boyd, W.C. (1950) op. cit., pp. 185

44. Montague, A. (1945) Man's Most Dangerous Myth: the Fallacy of Race, Columbia University Press, New York

45. The roots of racism, (1982) Progressive Labour Magazine, Brooklyn, New York Vol. 15, No.3

46. Montague, A. (1945) op. cit.

47. The roots of racism (1982) op. cit.

48. Morgan, E. (1975) American Slavery, American Freedom, W.W. Norton Company, New York

49. Bennet, L. (1966) Before the Mayflower. A History of the Negro in America 1619-1964 Penguin Books, Baltimore

50. Jordan, W. (1968) White Over Black: American Attitudes Toward the Negro, 1550-1812, Penguin books, Baltimore, MD

51. Boyer, R.O. and Morais, H.M. (1955) Labor's Untold Story, Cameron Associates, New York

52. Foster, W.Z. (1970) The Negro People in American History, International Publishers, New York

53. Haywood, H. (1934) Negro Liberation, International Publishers, New York

54. Foner, P. (1976) Organised Labor and the Black Worker, International Publishers, New York

55. Foster, W.Z. (1970) op. cit.

56. Haywood, H. (1934) op. cit.

57. Foner, P. (1976) op. cit.

58. Ibid.

59. Myrdal, G. (1944) An American Dilemma: The Negro Problem and Modern Democracy, Harper and Row, New York
60. Cherry, R (1978) Economic theories of racism, in D.M. Gordon (ed) Problems in Political Economy - an Urban Perspective, D.C. Heath and Company, Lexington, pp. 170-182
61. Myrdal, G. (1984) op. cit., pp. 508
62. Friedman, M. (1962) Capitalism and Freedom, University of Chicago Press, Chicago, pp. 110
63. Ibid., pp. 111
64. Becker, G. (1957) The Economics of Discrimination, University of Chicago Press, Chicago
65. The roots of racism (1982) op. cit.
66. Cherry, R. (1978) op. cit.
67. Reich, M. (1981) Racial Inequality: Political- Economic Analysis, Princeton University Press, Chicago
68. Silver, M. (1976) Employee taste for discrimination, wages and profits, in D. Mermelstein (ed) Economics: Mainstream Readings and Racial Critique, Random, New York
69. Tabb, W. (1971) Capitalism, colonialism, and racism, Review of Radical Political Economy Vol. 5, pp. 47-86
70. Cherry, R. (1973) Class struggle and the nature of the working class, Review of Radical Political Economy, Vol. 5, pp. 47-86
71. Reich, M. (1981) op. cit., pp. 147
72. Ibid., pp. 32
73. Ibid., pp. 32
74. Cooper, R., Steinhauer, M.J., Miller, W.H., Davis, R., Schatzkin, A. (1981) Racism, society and disease: an exploration of the social and biological mechanisms of differential mortality, International Journal of Health Services, Vol. 11, pp. 389-414
75. Susser, M. (1969) Ageing and the field of public health, in M.W. Riley, J.W. Rile, and M.E. Johnston. (eds) Ageing and Society, Russell Sage Foundation, New York, pp. 140-160
76. Binstock, R.H. and Shanas, E. (eds) (1976) Handbook of Ageing and the Social Sciences, Van Nostrand Reinhold Company, New York
77. Susser, M. (1969) op. cit.

78. Cooper, R. and Schatskin, A. (1982) The pattern of mass disease in the USSR, International Journal of Health Services, Vol. 12, pp. 459-480
79. Williams, R.A. (ed) Textbook of Black-Related Disease, McGraw-Hill, New York, pp. 4
80. Ibid., pp. 4
81. David, R.J. and Siegal, E. (1983) Decline in neonatal mortality rates, 1968-1977: better babies or better care?, Paediatrics, Vol. 71, pp. 531-540
82. Cassal, J. (1971) Summary of the major findings of the Evans County cardiovascular studies, Archives of Internal Medicine, Vol. 128, pp. 887-889
83. Tyroler, H.A. Hames, C.G, Krishan, I., Heyden, S. Cooper, G. and Cassel, J.C. (1975) Black-white differences in serum lipids and lipoproteins in Evans County, Preventive Medicine, Vol. 4, pp. 541-549
84. Coronary Heart Disease in black Populations, (A report of Two Symposia), American Heart Journal, Vol. 108, Part 2, September 1984
85. Cassal, J. (1971) op. cit.
86. Manton, K.G. (1982) Temporal and age variation of United States black/white cause-specific mortality differentials: a study of the recent changes in relative health status of the United States black population, The Gerontologist, Vol. 22, pp. 170-179
87. Strong, J.P., Restrepe, C. and Guzman, M., (1978) Coronary and Aortic Atherosclerosis in New Orleans, Laboratory Investigation, Vol. 39, pp. 364-371
88. Symposium: Coronary Heart Disease in black populations, Sponsored by the American Heart Association, San Diego, CA, March 5, 1983
89. Gillum, R.F. (1982) Coronary heart disease in black populations I, Mortality and Morbidity, American Heart Journal, Vol. 104, pp. 839-851
90. Gillum, R.F., Grant, D.T., (1982) Coronary heart disease in black populations II Risk Factors, American Heart Journal, Vol. 104, pp. 852-864

91. Mojonnier, M.L., Hall, Y., Berkson, D.M., Robinson, E., Wehters, B., Wannamaker, B., Moss,.D, Pardo, E., Stamler, J., Shekelle, R. and Raynor, W. (1980) Experience in changing food habits in hyperlipidemic men and women, Journal American Diet Association, Vol. 77, pp. 140-148

92. Marmot, M.G., Rose, G., Shipley, M. and Hamilton, P.J.S. (1978) Employment grade and coronary heart disease in British civil servants, Journal Epidemiology and Community Health, Vol. 32, pp. 244-249

93. Akinkugbe, O.O. and Bertrand E. (eds) (1975) Hypertension in Africa, Literamed, Lagos

94. Cooper, R. (1975) Blacks and hypertension, Urban Health, Vol. 4. pp. 9-14

95. Stamler, J., Stamler, R. and Pullman, T. (eds) (1964) The Epidemiology of Hypertension, Grune and Stratton, New York

96. Hypertension Detection and Follow-up Program Cooperative Group (1977) Race, education and prevalence of hypertension, American Journal of Epidemiology, Vol. 106, pp. 351-361

97. United States (1981) Hypertension in Adults 24-75 Years of Age, United States, 1971-1975, National Health Survey, US Department of Health and Human Services, Publ No. 81-1671, Hyattsville MD

98. Cooper, R. (1975) op. cit.

99. Trevisan, M., Ostrow, D., Cooper Liu K., Sparksand Okonek, A. (1983) Abnormal red blood cells in transport and hypertension, The People's Gas Company Study, Hypertension, Vol. 5, pp. 363-367

100. Canessa, M., Adragna, N., Solomon, H.S., Connoly, T.M. and Tosteson, D.C. (1980) Increased sodium-lithium countertransport, in red cells of patients with essential hypertension, New England Journal of Medicine, Vol. 302, pp. 772-776

101. Trevisan, M., Ostrow, D., Cooper, R., Sempos C., Stamler, J. (1984) Sex and Race Differences in sodium-Lithium Countertransport and Red Cell Sodium concentration, American Journal of Epidemiology, Vol. 120, pp. 537-541

102. United States (1983) Dietary source Data: United States, 1976-80, National Health Survey, Series II, No. 231, Department of Health and Human Services, Publ. No. 83-1681, Hyattsville, MD
103. Cooper, R. (1975) op. cit.
104. Keil, J.E., Tyroler, H.A., Sandifer and S.H., Boyle, E., (1977) Hypertension: effect of social class and racial admixture, The Results of a Cohort Study in the Black Population of Charleston, SC. American Journal of Public Health, Vol. 67, pp. 276-296
105. Ibid.
106. Moryiama, I., Krueger, D.E., and Stamler, J (1971) Cardiovascular Diseases in the United States, Harvard University Press, Cambridge
107. Ibid.
108. Cooper, R. et al (1981) op. cit.
109. Ibid.
110. Hammond, E.C. and Garfinkle, L. (1968) Changes in cigarette smoking, 1959-1965, American Journal of Public Health, Vol. 58, pp. 30-37
111. Lloyd, J.W. (1971) Long-term Mortality Study of Steelworkers, Journal of Occupational Medicines, Vol. 13, pp. 53-60
112. Miller, W.J. and Cooper, R. (1982) Rising cancer death rates among black men: the importance of occupation and social class, Journal National Medical Association, Vol. 74, pp. 253-258
113. Shekelle, R.B., Lepper, M., Liu, S., Maliza, C., Paynor, W.J.Jr., Rossof, A.H., Paul, O., Shryock, A.M. and Stamler, J. (1981) Dietary vitamin A and risk of cancer in the western electric study, Lancet, Vol. 2, pp. 1185-1190
114. United States (1983) op. cit.
115. Klebba, A.J. (1975) Homicide trends in the United States, 1900-74, Public Health Reports Vol. 90, pp. 195-204
116. Centerwall, B. (1984) Race, Socioeconomic Status, and Domestic Homicide: Atlanta, 1971-1972, American Journal of Public Health, Vol. 74, pp. 813-815

117.   Alcohol   use   and   alcoholism   among   black
        Americans, a review, in Harper, F D (ed),
        Alcoholism Treatment and Black Americans,
        Department   of   Health,   Education and
        Welfare,   National   Institute   on Alcohol
        Abuse   and   Alcoholism,   Rockville, M.D.,
        pp. 1-16 (1979)
118.   Cooper,   R.,   Liu,   K.,   Stamler, J.,
        Schoenberger,   J.A.,   Shekelle,   R.B.,
        Collette P.   and   Shekelle,   S.,   (1984)
        Prevalence   of   diabetes   hyperglycervia
        and   associated   cardiovascular   risk
        factors   in   blacks   and   whites, The
        Chicago   Heart   Association   Detection
        Project   in   Industry   American   Heart
        Journal, Vol. 108, pp. 827-833
119.   Ibid.
120.   Cooper, R. et al (1981) op. cit.
121.   Walker, A.R.P., (1980) The epidemiology of
        ischaemic   heart   disease   in   different
        ethnic populations in Johannesburg, South
        African Medical Journal Vol. 57, pp. 748-
        752
122.   Bradshaw, E. and Harrington, J.S. (1981) The
        cancer   problem   among   blacks: South
        Africa   in C. Mettlin, G.P. Murphy (eds),
        Cancer   Among   Black   Populations, Alan R
        Liss, New York, pp. 17-33
123.   Van Der Bergh, C. (1979) Smoking behaviour of
        White,   Black,   Coloured, and Indian South
        Africans,   South African Medical Journal,
        Vol. 55, pp. 975-979
124.   Reich, M. (1981) op. cit.
125.   Macmahon, B., Kovar, M.G. and Feldman, J.J.
        (1972)   Infant   mortality   ratio: socio-
        economic   factors,   Vital   Health
        Statistics, Series 22, No. 14
126.   Kessner,   D.M.,   Singer,   J.,   Kalk,   C.E.,
        Schelsinger, E.R.,(1973) Infant Death: An
        Analysis by Maternal Risk and Health Care
        National Academy of Sciences, Washington,
        DC
127.   Chase,   H.,   (1974)   Infant   Mortality and its
        concomitants,   1960-1972,   Medical   Care
        Vol. 15, pp. 662-667
128.   David,   R.   and   Reis,   J.,   (1984)   Race and
        infant mortality in US cities: effects
        of   race-specific   mortality   rates and
        black/white   differentials   (unpublished
        paper)

129. David, R.J. and Siegal, E. (1983) op. cit.
130. Reich, M. (1981) op. cit.
131. Cooper, R., Steinhauer, M., Schatzkin, A. and Miller, W., (1981) Improved mortality among US blacks, 1968-1978: The role of anti-racist struggle, International Journal of Health Services, Vol. 11, pp. 511-522
132. Aday, L.A., Anderson, R. and Fleming, G.V. (1980) Health Care in the United States: Equitable for Whom?, Sage Publications, Beverly Hills
133. Link, C.R., Long, S.H. and Settle, R.F. (1982) Access to medical care under medicaid: differentials by race, Journal Health Politics and Policy Law, Vol. 7, pp. 345-361
134. National Centre for Health Statistics (1965) Changes in Mortality Trends in England and Wales, 1931-1961, Public Health Service Publ. No. 1000, Series 3, No. 3, Washington DC
135. Cooper, R., (1981) Rising death rates in the Soviet Union; the impact of Coronary heart disease, New England Journal Medicine, Vol. 304, pp. 1259-1265
136. National Centre for Health Statistics (1973) Mortality Trends: Age, Colour and Sex, United States - 1950-1969, DHEW Publ. No (HRA) 74-1852, Rockville, MD
137. Moriyame, I.M., (1961) Preliminary observations on recent mortality trends, Public Health Reports, Vol. 76, 1956-1958
138. Cooper, R. and Sempos, C., (1984) Recent mortality patterns associated with economic development in eastern Europe and the USSR, Journal National Medical Association, Vol. 76, pp. 163-166
139. Cooper, R. and Schatzkin, A., (1982) Recent trends in coronary risk factors in the USSR, American Journal Public Health, Vol. 72, pp. 431-440
140. United States (1981) Artherosclerosis, 1981, Vol. 2, Report of Working Group on Artherosclerosis of the National Heart, Lung and Blood Institute, DHHS, Public Health Service, Bethesda, Sept, pp. 215
141. Preston, S.H. (1976) Mortality Patterns in National Populations, Academic Press, New York

142. Palloni, A. and Wyrick, R, (1982) Mortality decline in Latin America: changes in the structure of causes of deaths, 1950-1975, Social Biology, Vol. 28, pp 187-216
143. Aidoo, T.A. (1982) Rural health under colonialism and neo-colonialism: a survey of the Ghanaian experience, International Journal of Health Services, Vol. 12, pp. 637-657
144. Elling, R.H. (1981) The Capitalist world-system and international health, International Journal of Health Services, Vol. 11, pp. 21-51
145. Preston, S.H. (1976) op. cit.
146. Ibid.
147. Palloni, A. and Wyrick, R. (1982) op. cit.
148. Yunes, J. (1981) Evolution of infant mortality and proportional infant mortality in Brazil, World Health Statistics Quarterly, Vol. 34, pp. 200-219
149. Wood, C.H. (1982) The Political economy of infant mortality in San Paulo, Brazil, International Journal Health Services, Vol. 12, pp. 215-230
150. Moore, H.A., De La Cruz, E. and Vargas-Mendez, O. (1965) Diarrheal Disease in Costa Rica, American Journal of Epidemiology, Vol. 82, pp. 143-165
151. Preston, S.H. (1976) op. cit.
152. Paloni, A. and Wyrick, R. (1982) op. cit.
153. Gregory, J.W. and Piche, B. (1983) Inequality and mortality: demographic hypotheses regarding advanced and peripheral capitalism, International Journal Health Service, Vol. 13, pp. 343-351
154. Rodgers, G B, (1980) Income and inequality as determinants of mortality: an international cross-section analysis, Population Studies, Vol. 33, 2, pp. 343-351
155. Newland, K. (1982) Infant mortality and the health of societies, World Health Forum, Vol. 3, pp. 321-324
156. Palloni, A. and Wyrick, R. (1982) op. cit.

157. Gwatkin, D.R. (1980) Indications of change in developing country mortality trends: the end of an Era? Population Development Review, Vol. 6, pp. 615-644

158. Schatzkin, A (1983) Variation in Inpatient Racial Composition Among Acute-care Hospitals in New York State, (Abst), American Public Health Association Annual Convention

159. The Robert Woods Johnson Foundation (1978), Special Report: A New Survey on Access to Medical Care, No.1, The Robert Wood Johnson Foundation, Princeton, NJ

160. Aday, L. et al (1980) op. cit.

161. Apostolises, A.Y., Cutter, G., Kraus, J.F., Oberman, A., Blaszkowske, T., Borhani, N.O., Entwisle, G. (1980) Impact of hypertension information on high blood pressure control between 1973 and 1978, Hypertension, Vol. 2, pp. 708-713

162. Axtell, L.M. and Myers, M.H., (1978) Contrasts in survival of black and white cancer patients, 1960-1973, Journal National Institute, Vol. 60, pp. 1209-1214

163. Gwatkin, D.R.(1980) op. cit.

164. Leibel, R. (1977) Thanatology and medical economist, New England Journal Medicine, Vol. 305, pp. 667-670

165. Green, L., (1985) Health cutbacks and death with dignity: a right wing trend in medicine today, Radical Community Medicine, Spring, No. 21, pp. 20-26

166. Gildea, M. V. (1983) Euthanasia: A Review of the American Literature, Unpublished Thesis, Harvard University, March, 1983

167. Russel, O.R., (1975) Freedom to Die, Human Sciences Press, New York

168. Doctor's dilemma: treat or let die?, US News and World Report, pp. 53-56, 6 December 1982

169. Bewick, D.M. and Komarof, A. (1982) Cost effectiveness of lead screening, New England Journal of Medicine, Vol. 306, pp. 1392-1397

170. Mahaffey, K.R., Annest, J.L., Roberts, J. and Murphy, R.S., (1982) National estimates of blood lead levels: United States, 1976-1980, New England Journal of Medicine, Vol. 307, pp. 573-579

171. Schatzkin, A., (1984) The relationship of Inpatient racial composition and hospital closure in New York City, Medical Care, Vol. 22, pp. 379-387

172. Freis, J.F., (1980) Aging, natural death and the compression of mortality, New England Journal of Medicine, Vol. 303, pp. 130-135

173. Stead, E. (1982) Unsolved issues in medicine: geriatrics as a case in point, Journal of American Geriatrics Society, Vol. 30, pp. 231-234

174. Schatzkin, A., (1980) How long can we live? A more optimistic view of potential gains in life expectancy, American Journal of Public Health, Vol. 70, pp. 1199-1200

175. Gildea, M. (1983) op. cit.

176. Iglehart, J.K. (1982) Report on the Duke University Medical Center private sector conference, New England Journal of Medicine, Vol. 307, pp. 68-71

177. Rogers, D.E., Blendon, R.J. and Moloney, T.W. (1982) Who needs medicaid? New England Journal of Medicine, Vol. 307, pp. 13-18

178. Ibid.

179. Evans, R.W. (1983) Health care technology and the inevitability of resource allocation and rationing decisions, Journal of American Medical Medical Association, Vol. 249, pp. 2047-2061, 2208-2219

180. Lundberg, G.D. (1983) Rationing Human Life (Editorial) Journal of American Medical Association, Vol. 249, pp. 2223, 2224

181. Evans, R.W. (1983) op. cit., pp. 2217

182. Gildea, M. (1983) op. cit.

183. Wertham, F. (1966) The geranium in the window: the " euthanasia" murders, in F. Wertham A Sign for Cain, Macmillan, New York, pp. 602-641

Race, Disease and Health

184. Alexander, L. (1949) Medical science under dictatorship, New England Journal of Medicine, Vol. 241, pp. 39-47
185. Mitshcerlicj, R. and Mielke, G. (1949) Doctors in Infamy, Henry Schuman, Inc, New York
186. Wertham. F. (1966) op. cit.
187. Ibid.

Chapter 3

ETHNIC DIFFERENCES IN DISEASE - AN EPIDEMIOLOGICAL
PERSPECTIVE

Ranjit Bandaranyake

INTRODUCTION

Epidemiology is an extremely useful tool in
understanding disease mechanisms and causation. Its
methodology in common with a few other disciplines
lends itself to scientific research design. Its
products contribute to the rational planning of
health care services [1].
     Immigrant populations are of epidemiological
interest from several points of view. They may
play important roles in the importation and spread
of communicable disease. They may be susceptible
to environmental influences that would be innocuous
under normal circumstances for the indigenous
population. They may be exposed to stressful
situations which static populations do not
experience so frequently or so intensely. They
provide opportunities for the clarification of the
mechanism underlying unusual disease patterns noted
in particular places or particular ethnic
groups [2].
     The extent of the interaction between the
genetic endowment of an individual and the
environment in which he/she lives may be crucial in
the emergence of a specific disease. In ethnic
minority groups tuberculosis and mental illness for
example may have different degrees of genetic
component that influences susceptibility. The
ramifications of the physical and social
environments, which are important determinants of
health, are diverse and complicated. The
availability and use of health care facilities is
clearly a function of environment, human biology and
life-style [3,4].
     In this field of research, migrant groups
provide an interesting but by no means a
'captive' population. The usual dependence on
comparison in epidemiological studies may be less
meaningful in the context of isolated minority

groups for whom no accurate information is available
on disease patterns in their countries or
geographical districts of origin. Specific
features of a migrant group could confound the
issues further, for example, the more able, younger
and probably healthier persons may come in first,
later being joined by spouses and children who may
be much more susceptible to a variety of disease.

In general although migrant groups provide many
opportunities for research into aetiological
factors, the several pitfalls in study design and
interpretation of results must be borne in mind.
Well planned studies are essential however if one is
to provide a better understanding of disease
patterns and equitable service provision to these
ethnic minority groups in the community. Here,
ethnic minorities may be viewed as new immigrants
although it must be remembered as pointed out in
chapter one, by no means all such persons are new
in-migrants.

EPIDEMIOLOGICAL CONCEPTS

There are several useful definitions of epidemiology
of which the most widely applied is perhaps one
which refers to it as a method of studying the
distribution and determinants (or aetiology) of
disease in human populations. It is in essence
however more than merely a method in that it has all
the basic characteristics of a science, such as
specific theoretical structure, distinctive
methodology, recognised application and an
identifiable domain of discourse. One of several
other definitions of this science is from a paper by
Professor Lilianfeld, in which he describes
epidemiology as "a way of reasoning about disease in
human populations, using biological inferences
derived from both observations and experiment" [5].
Human populations or specific sub-groups are
observed from a view point of health and disease and
sometimes an intervention is made in an attempt to
alter the natural history of a disease, hopefully
for the better. The intervention study is now a
recognised type of investigation in modern
epidemiology [6,7]. As an essential pre-requisite
to both observation and intervention one attempts
to define, as precisely as possible, both the
population of interest and the disease under
consideration. Where circumstances permit one

incorporates a scientific design into this intervention in order to extrapolate the results to the wider population.

Experimentation within human populations is ethically unjustifiable in most, if not all, situations. Indeed, this is often now so even within animal populations. However, there are still a few circumstances in which experimentation in the pure sense using random control designs is acceptable. These can sometimes include the trials designed to test new drugs and vaccines as well as new management regimes within the sphere of medical care although not all would agree with this. More importantly, at least from the epidemiological viewpoint, use is made of certain naturally occurring situations which lend themselves to experimental design. These studies usually focus on environmental changes, either naturally occurring or man-made, such as fluoridation of water supplies, or the availability of soft or hard water and their relationship with disease incidence. More interestingly, some studies focus both on environmental change and behaviour or life-style modification. These are predominantly the migrant studies, and it is this category which will be considered in some detail below.

The human organism, both singly and collectively, is exposed to the total environment and its fluctuations. Minor changes are easily coped with under normal circumstances by healthy individuals through a process known as the compensatory response [8]. No ill-effects are expected from such changes, none are generally found. Indeed these minor alterations of the status-quo are regarded not merely as part and parcel of everyday living but as an essential element for proper bodily functioning. Major changes in the environment can pose problems for the human body, particularly if such changes occur frequently over long periods of time or continuously over a short span. Although there is much individual variation in response and effect, all human beings exhibit a 'break point' beyond which the compensatory non-destructive response fails, and derangement of bodily functions results. This is invariably expressed as either physical or psychological disease, or, as is becoming increasingly apparent, a combination of both; the so-called psychosomatic manifestations.

Ethnic Differences in Disease

The environment in relation to health and
disease is best defined as the totality of external
influences, natural and man-made, that impinge on
man and affect his well-being. It includes the
physical environment, the microbiological
environment and the social environment. The
importance of this last component is often not
appreciated by the medical profession when looking
at disease causation and intervention [9,10]. It
comprises social, economic, cultural and religious
norms which may be crucial in the way in which
people look upon health and illness and their use of
the health services. These factors also
undoubtedly influence behaviour which is quite
obviously associated with many of the diseases of
modern times.
The physical environment has been and probably
still remains, at least for some groups, the most
important determinant of health and disease. The
vast improvement in the health of the population in
the Western World is, undoubtedly due to
environmental, economic and social changes
particularly in the area of nutrition and sanitation
beginning in the last quarter of the 19th Century.
Although any further breakthrough in the type of
disease picture now seen in developed countries
would most probably be through behaviour
modification, there remain population sub-groups
which may benefit even today by attention to the
physical environment. This applies not only to the
ethnic minority groups but also to vast numbers of
indigenous families who are disadvantaged,
unemployed, and occupy unhealthy dwellings without
even some of the basic amenities, and to certain
industrial or occupational situations.
The major advantage in identifying detrimental
environmental factors in relation to disease in
ethnic minority groups is the possible alteration of
these factors with limited dependence on behavioural
change necessary to demonstrate some benefit.
Benefits that accrue, for instance ante-natal care
and communicable disease control, need not
necessarily be confined to the minority groups for
they may be of value to all sectors of society.
Two important determinants of health, namely the
environment and behaviour have so far been
mentioned. It need hardly be explained that there
is an interaction between these two determinants,
and it is this correlation which is probably the
crucial factor which needs to be taken into account

when one attempts to explain the incidence of disease in migrant groups. There are, however, two other determinants which must be considered separately and in combination with both the environment and behaviour. These are genetic endowment and availability and use of health care facilities.

The extent of the interaction between genetic endowment and the environment is of particular interest in the emergence of specific diseases. The true contribution of each of these determinants to the emergence of a disease is also of great importance. It is for example often stated, without adequate evidence, that Caucasian populations have a genetically inbuilt resistance to pulmonary tuberculosis. This implies that other non-Caucasian groups do not possess this resistance and indeed may have an increased susceptibility to the disease. The reverse may be true for dental caries and ischaemic health disease although recent evidence from developing countries indicated that the incidence of the latter condition is increasing in affluent sub-groups residing mainly in larger cities. Mental illness, which is now being diagnosed increasingly among ethnic minority groups, is another such category which is said to have a strong genetic component which lies dormant until environmental changes produce sufficient stress to make these conditions apparent. There are obvious dangers in carrying this argument too far and equating genetic pre-dispositions with racial characteristics. The fallacies that can then be derived have already been referred to by Richard Cooper (chapter two) but to ignore possible genetic factors could be equally unwise. The following diagram (Figure 3.1) indicates the importance of genetic and environmental factors for particular diseases.

The availability and use of health care facilities have obvious implications for minority groups both in the early detection of disease, as in screening for cancer of the cervix, and in optimal care of certain groups such as pregnant mothers and their utilisation of antenatal clinics. Early contact with health care providing agencies may also have an impact on the natural history of the disease in question. It is not intended here to enlarge on the various shortcomings of the British National Health Service (NHS) in relation to these minority groups as these have already been well-documented

Figure 3.1: The Genetic and Environmental Relationship with Disease

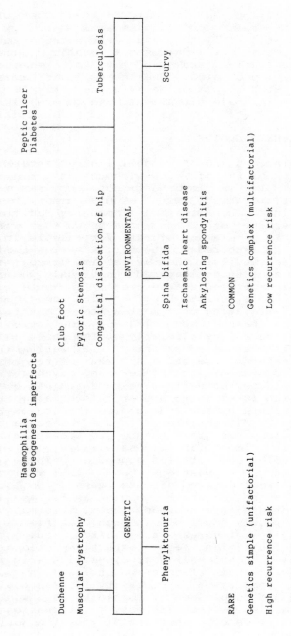

elsewhere [11,12].   Suffice   it   to   say   that the
service   does   break   down   in   several   situations
possibly   due   to   a   lack   of   understanding of the
cultural   and behavioural patterns of ethnic groups,
lack   of   communication,   and even at times a relative
lack   of   basic   provision.   The Inverse Care Law so
aptly   highlighted   by Tudor Hart in the early 1970s
may well apply in these situations even today [13].

MIGRANT AND ETHNIC GROUPS

Migrant   populations are of epidemiological interest
from   several   points   of   view although as noted in
chapter   1,   it   is   important   not   to   view new
immigrants   as   identical   with   ethnic   minorities.
Studies done in the Department of Community Medicine
at   the   University   of   Leeds   have shown that even
within   the   UK   people who migrate for example from
Scotland   to   England reduce their risk status for a
variety of diseases [14]. The reverse is, of course,
true   for   those less enlightened individuals who go
North   in search of a pure 'wee drop'.   The mere act
of   boarding   an   aircraft   from   any less developed
country   and   emigrating   to   most Western countries
would   likewise   reduce   the   risk   of   contacting a
variety   of diseases, particularly of the infectious
type.   It   will   also reduce the risk of perinatal,
infant   and   maternal   death.   But what of the non-
communicable   diseases;   the cancers and psychiatric
illnesses?   To date, no definitive research has been
published   which attempts to answer this question in
relation to Asian and West Indian minority groups in
Britain.   The   difficulties   to   be   overcome in
mounting   a   study   of   this nature are such that it
would   make   it   almost   an   impossibility.   By and
large   epidemiological   studies depend on comparison
of   well-defined   populations   and   the   various
incidences   of well-defined disease states.   Obvious
deficiencies   exist   on   both   counts   as far as the
country   of   origin is concerned.   Basic information
systems   are   poorly developed in such countries and
even   mortality   figures   are   often   suspect.
Diagnostic   facilities   and   expertise   too are
available   to   a much lesser degree, particularly in
the   more   rural   areas of these countries.   In such
circumstances   comparison of mortality figures could
be misleading and comparison of morbidity data would
almost   certainly   be   meaningless.   International
Mortality Statistics published annually by the World

Health Organization (WHO) give only a broad indication and are of use mainly in identifying secular trends within countries. They do not form an adequate basis for comment when comparing less-developed countries with, for example, England and Wales. Ad hoc surveys done by well-trained epidemiologists and joint efforts between countries are required for any useful studies of this nature.

This is not to say that studies of other migrant populations are not available. Indeed there are several studies producing valuable epidemiological information on both the Japanese migrants to the United States and the Israeli migrants returning to their 'native land' during the period after the Second World War. These studies have shown that, in spite of the often overriding effects of environmental change and behaviour modification particularly in relation to dietary habits, the genetic influences remain, and in adequately designed surveys can indeed be recognised. More interestingly, one study which focused on the increased incidence of coronary heart disease within a Japanese migrant population in the United States as compared to the Japanese in Japan demonstrated that even in a situation of higher overall incidence of this disease, the sub-group which retained its cultural pattern and lifestyle and thereby had social support from its own members had a much lesser risk of both developing the condition and dying from it [15]. These results were obtained after controlling for all other known major risk factors such as smoking and hypertension [16,17]. Conversely links between disease incidence and social 'stress' have been well documented [18-20]. There are lessons to be learned from such findings, that may well apply to the Asian and West Indian migrant groups in this country, at least amongst first generation migrants at any rate.

Immigrant populations can play important roles in the importation and spread of communicable disease. In general this statement is true, although much unnecessary blame has been attributed to such groups in the past and, likewise, much misplaced concern expressed by the media about the possibilities of both importation and spread of such disease. In order fully to appreciate the situation it is necessary to differentiate between infection and disease. Consider, for example, pulmonary tuberculosis. Evidence suggests that the overall prevalence of this condition is higher among

Asian minority groups [21]. New immigrants may probably enter the country with the infection but this can only be detected by special, non-routine investigations. Once in this country environmental stresses may play an important part in the breakdown of the body's defences, and the disease could manifest itself. This is the simplest picture that can be drawn, but it is not necessarily the true sequence of events. It is equally likely that the infection itself is acquired in the crowded, often poorly heated and ventilated houses they live in, at least initially soon after arrival. Poor dietary intake and other social stresses too, undoubtedly, contribute to the emergence of the disease. There is often also some delay in seeking medical care. The disease itself is, however, not peculiar to the Asian minority groups. For example, recent figures show that in the Airedale Health District, part of which includes the Bradford Metropolitan local government district, the prevalence of pulmonary tuberculosis is high, and disproportionately so in the Caucasian population. From an historical angle we know that Irish immigrants to England commonly suffered from this disease in spite of climatic conditions being little different and dietary intake no worse than in the famine-stricken farming areas of Ireland during the potato blight.

Most diseases of the communicable variety, particularly the enteric fevers such as typhoid may occasionally be found within Asian sub-groups in England. Some acquire the disease when returning to England after a brief visit to their home country. Others may be unidentified carriers of the disease and commonly transmit it to members usually of the same community. In the existing situation of comparatively high standards of sanitation at least for the vast majority of the indigenous population however, epidemic spread of these diseases is rare. The last typhoid outbreak in the UK, in Aberdeen, was caused by contaminated corned beef from South America which had no links whatsoever with ethnic minority groups. Nevertheless, the fact cannot be ignored that the prevalence of most of these conditions is generally higher among ethnic minority groups and, as such, they form a potential pool of infectivity which would be of greater concern in a less hygienic environment. The root cause may be disadvantage in terms of social conditions and employment opportunities.

THE LOCAL SCENE

In the Bradford Health District, the 1981 census
illustrates that 6.7% of persons resident are known
to have been born outside the UK in the New
Commonwealth and Pakistan (NCWP) compared with
approximately 4% for the whole UK (this figure of
6.7% increases to 11.2% if country of birth of the
head of the household is taken into account) [22].
Nearly one-half of Bradford's NCWP population is
under 16 years of age, and there are fewer than a
thousand pensioners with origins in that part of the
world. This pattern is bound to change with time
but it will be many years before the demographic
structure of the ethnic minority group approximates
to that of the local population. At least in this
respect the ethnic minority group cannot be included
in the category of high NHS resource consumers
(children and the elderly).
    There is a variety of health issues concerning
this minority group and no attempt will be made even
to list all of them. Neither will there be an
attempt to describe the total health profile of the
predominantly Asian sub-group. The following
sections are intended only to indicate some of the
areas of concern, and in particular relate them to
epidemiological research in progress or planned in
this district.

Tuberculosis
Up to the end of 1981 approximately 75% of all
tuberculosis in Bradford occurred in Asian
immigrants. The picture has changed somewhat in
1982 due entirely to one epidemic associated with a
local pub in which 41 persons, all of Caucasian
origin, presented with the disease or were traced,
and of these 34 had not been protected with BCG
vaccine [23]. During the late 1970s there was a
general increase in notifications in Asians in the
age group 15-29 , with a slight excess in females.
This female excess was due mainly to the
disproportionate number of cases amongst Pakistani
women. From 1980 onwards there has been a slight
change in these trends. Not only have the number
of cases of tuberculosis in young adults of Asian
origin decreased but the proportion of notifications
from the Asian group has also been reduced. Table
3.1 summarises these observations. It is too early
to be certain of the permanency of these trends,

but if they continue it would be an indication of
the success of efforts in Bradford aimed at
preventing and treating the disease in the minority
groups. It also emphasises the fact that the
disease in the indigenous population is not confined
to, for example, social outcasts and alcoholics, but
could easily occur in non-immunised young people
unless high immunity levels are maintained. Indeed,
as mentioned already, in the adjacent Airedale
Health District over the past two years at least,
the number of notifications from the indigenous
population has increased with an appreciable
proportion falling in the younger age groups.

Table 3.1: Notification of Tuberculosis in
Bradford 1976-1982

Age 15-29 years				Age 0-14 years	
Year					
	Male		Female		
	White	Asian	White	Asian	White	Asian
1976	6	40	7	41	2	3
1977	3	29	0	35	3	9
1978	5	37	2	43	3	7
1979	5	30	6	50	6	7
1980	5	33	6	26	1	10
1981	2	22	2	28	2	4
1982	18	21	17	14	3	11

Source: Bradford Health Authority

The other point of interest in support of what has
already been referred to earlier is the fact that
only a small percentage of the disease seems to be
actually imported. The breakdown of a quiescent
lesion accounts only for a small proportion of the
total incidence. Arrival in this country with an
infection but no evidence of disease which later
breaks down by a process of indigenous exacerbation
in which with fresh exposure to the bacillus may
play an important part. The majority of cases
however appear to be acquired after arrival in this
country, probably as a result of enhanced
susceptibility, poor environmental conditions,
mainly overcrowding and damp housing, and contact
with infected relatives. There is however little
agreement as to the relative importance of these

various modes of origin [24,25]. In Bradford Health
District there has recently been much interest in a
research exercise involving disease mapping and
tuberculosis has been selected as one of the first
diseases to be investigated. For the years 1979 to
1982 all notifications, numbering close to 500 have
been denoted on a large scale map as precisely as
possible. Some interesting clusters have been
observed in the predominantly high immigrant areas,
and demographic and environmental indices such as
ethnic group, age structure, and type of housing,
correlate well with these areas of high incidence.

The idea that the incidence of tuberculosis is
higher in Asians just because of their race is a
myth, as race is purely a social concept with no
biological meaning and does not play any role in the
genetic susceptibility to disease. The fact
that Asians tend to aggregate in the lower socio-
economic classes, and to live in some of the worst
housing areas and in overcrowded conditions increase
the likelihood of their having or contracting the
disease. Because it is an infectious disease
tuberculosis is spread more effectively under
certain environmental conditions as found in the
inner city areas of Bradford.

Gastro-intestinal Infections

It is generally accepted that the type of infections
found in the Asian sub-group in this country varies
from that found among the indigenous
population [26]. Scrutiny of disease notifications
would indicate that sporadic cases of typhoid and
paratypoid occur predominantly in the minority
groups. This also applies to certain organisms such
as shigella flexneri and shigella dysenteriae which
are commonly imported into this country from the
Indian sub-continent by residents returning from
holiday. In the case of shigella sonnei however the
picture is entirely different. This particular
strain is endemic in the UK and in the event of an
outbreak such as the one seen in Bradford during
1983/4 one would expect an equal representation
proportionately of cases from both the Asian and
Caucasian groups. Of a total of almost 1400 positive
isolations from the faeces of cases and contacts,
one would expect 10%, that is 140 cases among
Asians, as approximately 10% of the population of
Bradford Metropolitan District is of Asian origin.

If however one were to consider the fact that over
70% of such positives were from children between the
ages of 3 and 12 years, and that the age structure
of this Asian sub-group is heavily biased in favour
of these age groups, the number of cases expected
should be in the order of 15%. Furthermore, if
allowance is also made for the fact that the
majority of this population live in the most overcrowded and least modernised parts of the city, and
some importance is attached to environmental factors
such as bad housing in the spread of the disease, an
even higher proportion of positive cases may be
expected. There were in fact only 70 cases of
dysentery amongst Asians and most of these were in
children from one special school for the mentally
subnormal. There was ample opportunity for spread
within the Asian households as this infection would
certainly have been introduced through the children
in the above-mentioned school. There was, however,
little or no evidence of spread within households.
One might argue that the small numbers were due to
under-notification amongst this group. This is a
possibility, but cannot entirely explain the
deficit. It could well be that good personal
hygiene which is of paramount importance in the
context of this disease and is a way of life both
from a cultural and religious point of view had in
fact resulted in keeping numbers of cases to a
minimum within this population.

The Common Infectious Diseases of Childhood
These include the notifiable diseases such as
measles, whooping cough and diphtheria, as well as
those that are not statutorily notifiable, such as
rubella. The following comments apply mainly to the
former category.
     Meaningful comparisons of the incidence of
these notifiable diseases between districts is not
possible due to differences in the awareness of the
importance of notification among doctors. The
possible exceptions to this would be the more
serious conditions such as diphtheria which are
unlikely to go unnotified. Notifications are,
however, a useful method of observing secular trends
within districts as the inaccuracies in the figures
tend to matter less for this purpose.
     For most of these conditions the position in
Bradford reflects the national picture, but at a
somewhat higher level. The classic example is

measles. This disease which has a high incidence in less-developed countries also shows a high case fatality rate. This is acknowledged to be due to the concomitant poor nutritional state in the younger age group and their inability to develop both an adequate resistance to infection and antibodies to fight the disease once established. Over a 12 week period commencing 1st April 1983, more than a third of all notifications of measles in West Yorkshire have been from the Bradford Health District. The immunisation uptake is known to be poor at 58% but not very different from the other districts in the region. Figures for the uptake of this vaccine by Asian children are not available at present. The high incidence is unlikely to be due to the higher proportion of Asian children in Bradford, and the case-fatality rate which is extremely low could be due to an improved nutritional status although higher standards of medical care may also play a part.

A continuing research project in Bradford is based on a novel technique to study immunisation uptake for a variety of diseases. This has utilised the life-tables method applied to various birth cohorts of children. The information is available from the computerised vaccination and immunisation recall system although extraction and interpretation of this data are not a simple matter. What the study has shown so far is that there is a reasonable uptake of immunisation by the Asian ethnic minority group but within this group various sub-groups show vast differences in uptake. The Indians having the highest figures in general, (higher even than the Caucasian population) and the mixed sub-groups (that is half-Asian and half-Negro) have the lowest for all types of childhood immunisations.

A useful extension of this study which is being envisaged is to link the disease notification rates with the uptake of vaccine within these birth cohorts analysed by ethnic group. This could emphasise the importance of the immunisation procedure while pinpointing the population at highest risk for further action, for example, by health visitor input to promote immunisation.

Coronary Heart Disease

The initial reaction to the mention of this disease which is the major killer in the middle aged and elderly groups in most affluent countries is that it does not concern ethnic minority groups [27]. In Bradford there is now some evidence to show that this assumption may not be correct.

In the UK as a whole the mortality rate has risen over the past 30 years in both sexes and at all ages [28]. In the age group 45 to 64, coronary disease accounts for 40% of deaths in men and 10% in women. Females however lose their resistance to this condition soon after the menopause. Death rates are also higher in the lower social classes [29].

Table 3.2: Ischaemic Heart Disease Mortality – 1981 Comparison of Bradford and England and Wales

AGE (years)	35–44		45–54		55–64		over 65	
	M[a]	F[b]	M	F	M	F	M	F
England & Wales	0.53	0.08	2.61	0.46	6.98	2.00	20.75	12.47
Bradford	0.74	0.29	3.29	0.66	8.08	2.47	26.13	15.91

[a] Male
[b] Female

Source: Bradford Health Authority

It may be seen from Table 3.2 that for both sexes and over all age groups for the year 1981 mortality rates for Ischaemic Heart Disease were higher in Bradford when compared with England and Wales as a whole [30,31]. These rates have not been standardised for social class which may have an influence on their distribution. There is reason to believe that the rate is disproportionately high for incidence as well as mortality in the younger male Asians in Bradford. When dealing with small numbers as in this case, data collected over a number of years needs to be looked at for meaningful analysis. A retrospective study in Bradford which is attempting to throw some light on the situation is currently being initiated. It is tempting to speculate at this stage on the possible causes, such as a known higher cigarette consumption among young Asian males, a change in Western style diet and possible higher levels of stress, but without firm evidence such speculation would be very misleading.

Ethnic Differences in Disease

Environmental Hazards - Lead

Recent publicity in Bradford and Airedale Health Districts on the possible dangers to the health of primary school children due to higher than acceptable levels of lead in playground dust has resulted in a major study being launched to screen the primary school population. The method used is based on detection using fingerprick samples of blood of a substance named erythrocyte protoporphyrin which is linked to the synthesis of haemoglobin. Raised levels of this substance which can be measured using a portable machine in the field indicates either a high blood level or iron deficiency anaemia.

Lead is a multi-source problem and is of greatest danger to the younger child and the unborn infant. Although the ingestion of playground dust could be significant, the main hazards exist in the home where there may be old lead-based paint peeling off due to neglect, and lead pipes which can increase appreciably the lead content of drinking water left standing overnight. Based on these facts, the focus is again on the Asian minority groups in the district, even without taking into account the much publicised problem of lead-based eye-make-up (Surma) and tonic preparations containing lead. Some of these minority groups occupy a large proportion of the inner city houses which have all or some of the hazards referred to above. They may not be able to keep the dwellings in good repair due to financial difficulties, and unless communication is adequate and appropriate, they will not realise both the dangers that exist and what help is available in terms of grants from the Local Authority to replace lead pipes and the like. Furthermore, it is these very families who have more children in the younger age groups and a higher fertility rate. The younger children have a higher worm infestation rate which itself could cause anaemia as well as result in pica or abnormal eating habits, including chewing painted surfaces.

Initial results of the pilot survey have confirmed the above suspicions. Those children who have so far been identified as having high levels of blood lead and/or anaemia are children of Asian parents, and further investigations are now proceeding both with a view to screening other members of these families, particularly siblings, and investigating housing conditions. There has been an assurance of all feasible remedial measures

Table 3.3: Bradford Health District Stillbirths and
Infant Deaths by Social Class 1979-1981
(Rates per 1,000 total births.   Actual numbers in
parenthensis)

Social Class	Non-Handicapping Conditions		Handicapping Conditions	
	Asian	Non-Asian	Asian	Non-Asian
I and II	7.2(3)	5.9(13)	–	3.6(8)
III	16.3(22)	11.0(78)	14.1(19)	3.7(26)
IV and V	23.2(76)	24.3(71)	20.0(65)	10.6(31)

Source: Specialist in Community Medicine (Child
Health) Bradford Health Authority.

being available from both health and local
authorities.   One obvious difficulty is of course,
the fact that we are here dealing mainly with
private, usually owner-occupied or privately-rented
houses, and action from the local authority could be
limited to advice regarding re-painting, once the
lead pipes have been replaced. Air-borne pollution,
of course, may be subject to wider environmental
control.

Perinatal and Infant Mortality
This is the final category of concern, and probably
the most difficult to deal with in spite of much
available information and expertise.   No attempt
will therefore be made to paint a comprehensive
picture but rather to highlight some interesting
observations over the recent years.

It has always been apparent that both perinatal
and infant mortality rates are higher in ethnic
minority groups, particularly the Asian sub-groups.
This may be seen in the Bradford Health District,
but recent trends give cause for optimism [32].
Rates are falling particularly for perinatal
mortality although one must be aware of the
fluctuations due mainly to the small numbers
involved.

Using routinely collected maternity information
it is possible to relate perinatal and infant deaths
to total or live births for comparative purposes,

and referral to base population figures is fortunately not necessary. For example, if one wishes to compare still-births and infant deaths by social class for Asian and non-Asian groups, controlling for handicapping and non-handicapping conditions, basic information on the social class of mothers based on the occupation of their husbands could be extracted from the records (Table 3.3).

The validity of this comparison in terms of social class is open to question, and it cannot be defended totally. It does, however, show that for non-handicapping conditions although the social class gradient is apparent there is no significant difference between the Asian and non-Asian groups. This is not so for handicapping conditions where there is a marked difference in social classes III, and IV and V combined. These handicapping conditions include all cardiovascular, central nervous system, and other organ defects, as well as the multiple physical defects, and have remained excessive over the years in the ethnic minority groups.

CONCLUSION

It must be emphásised that this chapter has dwelt mainly on the situations and health issues that are currently being investigated in Bradford Health District. There are several other areas that have not been mentioned, psychiatric illness being one of note. Differences in disease occur also in reverse, some conditions being much less common in ethnic minority groups, for instance most cancers, chronic bronchitis, and so on which have not been referred to. Information for epidemiological studies is available from routinely collected data but may need to be supplemented by specific ad-hoc surveys. Information sources are several and not necessarily confined to that available in the NHS. Much useful data relating particularly to the denominator population and its characteristics are available from the Local Authority and it is in everybody's interest to establish close links between authorities and develop an integrated information system. The development of such co-operative/collaborative studies should perhaps become a major priority for professionals in the future.

REFERENCES

1. Knox, E.G. (ed) (1979) Epidemiology in Health Care Planning, Oxford University Press, Oxford
2. McMahon, B., and Pugh, T.F. (1970) in Epidemiology: Principles and Methods, Churchill Livingstone, London
3. Lalonde, M. (1974) A New Perspective on the Health of Canadians, Government of Canada, Ottawa
4. Long, A.F. (1984) Research into Health and Illness, Gower, Aldershot
5. Lilienfeld, D.E. (1978) Definitions of epidemiology, American Journal of Epidemiology, Vol. 107, pp. 87-90
6. Knox, E. (1979) op. cit.
7. Long, A. (1984) op. cit.
8. Catalona, R. (1979) Health, Behaviour and the Community, Pergamon Press, Oxford
9. Lalonde, M (1974) op. cit.
10. Long, A. (1984) op. cit.
11. Donovan, J. (1984) Ethnicity and health: a research review, Social Science and Medicine, Vol. 19, pp. 663-670
12. Rathwell, T. (1984) General practice, ethnicity and health services, Social Science and Medicine, Vol. 19, pp. 663-670
13. Hart, J.T. (1971) The inverse care law, Lancet, Vol. 1 pp. 405-412
14. McDonnell, H. (1973) The Mortality Rates of Migrants between England, Wales and Scotland, M.Sc. Thesis, Department of Community Medicine, Leeds University
15. Marmot, M. (1975) Acculturation and Coronary Heart Disease in Japanese Americans, Ph.D. dissertation, University of California
16. Ibid.
17. Cassel, J. (1976) The contribution of the social environment to host resistance, American Journal of Epidemiology, Vol. 104, pp. 107-123

18. Holmes, T. (1956) Multidiscipline studies of tuberculosis, in P.J. Sparer (ed) Personality Stress and Tuberculosis, New York, International Universities Press, Chapter 6

19. Dunham, H.W. (1961) Social structure and mental disorders: competing hypotheses of explanation, Milbank Memorial Fund, Vol. 39, pp. 259-311

20. Mishler, E.G. and Scotch, N.A. (1963) Socio-cultural factors in the epidemiology of schizophrenia: a review, Psychiatry, Vol. 26, pp. 315-351

21. Donovan, J. (1984) op. cit.

22. City of Bradford Metropolitan Council, Census Bulletin Series Multicultural Bradford, 1981

23. Hill, J.D. and Stevenson, D.K. (1983) Tuberculosis in unvaccinated children, adolescents and young adults: a city epidemic, British Medical Journal, Vol. 282, pp. 1471-1473

24. Office of Population Censuses and Surveys Census 1981, Small Area Statistics, Bradford and Airedale (OPCS), Provisional estimates of population

25. Office of Population Censuses and Surveys Monitor DH 81/4. Deaths by Cause, 1980, and OPCS S.D. 25 forms Bradford and Airedale

26. Johnson, M. (1984) Ethnic minorities and health: a review, Journal Royal College of Physicians, Vol. 18, pp. 228-230

27. Qureshi, B. (1981) Transcultural medicine, Pulse Magazine, October 29, November 5, November 12 (supplements)

28. Townsend, P. and Davidson, N. (1982) Inequalities in Health: The Black Report, Penguin, Harmondsworth

29. Ibid.

30. OPCS (1981) op. cit.

31. OPCS (1980) op. cit.

32. Ibid.

Chapter 4

THE POLITICS OF ETHNIC MINORITY HEALTH STUDIES

Maggie Pearson

INTRODUCTION - RESEARCH AND POLICIES ON RACE AND
HEALTH

In recent years, increasing attention has been
focused on ethnic minorities in Britain. The
development of Community Relations Councils,
professional training and initiatives in welfare and
education services have been reflected in a growth
of research, academic journals and institutions. A
quick glance at any public appointments page in one
of the major daily or weekly papers will reveal
several posts for 'specialists' to work with, or
research on ethnic minorities.

This rapid growth of what many aptly call 'the
Race Relations Industry' [1,2] has been the subject
of considerable debate, controversy, resentment and
anger. Many white people feel that their needs are
being neglected whilst 'these blacks with bleeding
hearts (sic)' receive disproportionate attention and
finance. Black radicals and critics view such
initiatives as, at best, window dressing; or at
worst intentional yet subtle, oppressive measures to
contain and defuse black dissent in which reforms
are implemented by agencies of a double edged state
which also colludes with, and participates in,
social relations and racist ideologies which produce
discrimination and reproduce disadvantage [3].

To many independent observers, watching from
the sidelines, the controversy often appears
incomprehensible. Why is it that people who stand
to gain from studies and institutes designed to
expose and publicise their problems, difficulties
and disadvantage object to them so vigorously? How
can it be racist to expose discrimination and
disadvantage, and advocate measures to ameliorate
its effects? Surely measures to redress the balance
of inequity are only to be welcomed?

Some of the resentment and cynicism stems from
the growing feeling that more and more academic
research which has amassed ample evidence of racial

discrimination and disadvantage [4] has produced no tangible results or committed and positive action to attack the fundamental roots of the situation - racism. This divorce of research from committed action is understandably viewed with increasing suspicion and hostility by black people who are the objects of more and more research. The established approach to science, based on the need for empirical, 'objective' information and 'facts' to prove the case implies a view that society is innocent of racism until proved guilty. For black people more 'objective' evidence is unnecessary: racism is an indisputable and oppressive force in their lives. The emphasis on well-documented research as a prerequisite for change is seen as a delaying tactic and an effective decoy from the root cause of their problems: racism.

The term 'ethnic' is used intentionally in this paper, for it is precisely within that culturalist framework which hinges fundamentally on the notion of 'ethnicity' that data on black people's health have largely been researched and collected. This data and its underlying philosophy have in turn informed policies and service initiatives which have been particularly directed at black people. By insisting on a focus on 'cultural differences', the cultural pluralists deny the centrality of race and racism in structuring black people's experience.

Since the 1960s, there have been policies and research on race and health. Early approaches addressed themselves to the health problems of 'immigrant' populations, emphasising imported, exotic and infectious disease for which a particular medical officer of health may be given special responsibility. This approach was the precursor of a now growing interest in, and awareness of 'ethnic' differences in morbidity and mortality which has been the subject of several recent professional conferences and 'special' initiatives and policies in the health service for ethnic minorities (as discussed in chapter 3).

The Rickets Campaign launched by the Department of Health and Social Security (DHSS) in 1981 was directed specifically at the 'Asian' community. In June 1984 the DHSS launched a new Asian Mother and Baby Campaign which stemmed from the previous Rickets Campaign. Many health authorities specifically vaccinate all Asian babies with BCG, as protection against tuberculosis: or specifically screen Asian and Far Eastern women for Hepatitis 'B' virus [5].

The majority of these 'special' health initiatives have met with fierce criticism from some of the communities which they purport to help. The objections are that the policies and the research that has informed them are racist because they focus exclusively on black problems without critically reflecting on the centrality of racism in structuring black people's health and experience of health services. Moreover, the research agendas have been defined by professionals and their perceived priorities of health problems, which are not necessarily those of black people using the Health Service. The emphasis on black pathology in increased morbidity and mortality is mirrored by an emphasis on perceived cultural deficits which policies have presumed to try to rectify.

In this chapter it is intended to present a review and critique of 'white race relations/ ethnicity' sociology on the one hand, and the politics and 'victim-blaming' ideology of medicine on the other, and show how these articulate and reinforce each other. It is argued that a focus on black and ethnic minority people often defines their cultures as pathological and pathogenic, resistant to the change which is necessary for them to adopt 'healthy' habits and lives.

RACE/ETHNIC RELATIONS STUDIES: WHO/WHAT IS THE PROBLEM?

Central to the controversy and criticism surrounding race relations/ethnic minority studies is their explicit focus, the implied definition of the nature of race relations, and the identity of the 'problem'. This issue is one of fundamental importance, being reflected in the way that findings and interpretations relate to policies and professional practice. Whilst recognising the pitfalls of over generalising from a variety and spectrum of approaches into a few 'schools of thought', there is a dichotomy between studies which take culture as their focus, and those which address themselves to the political sphere of power relations, seeing racism as part of the class relations of capitalism [6].

It is not the intention of this paper to undertake a detailed review of that controversy, since this has been discussed by Cooper (chapter 2), and of the various elements which have contributed to the 'success' of the focus on culture in attaining dominance and influence. What follows here is a summary of the major critique of the particular tradition of 'ethnic relations' sociology which has been a significant influence in shaping and informing public policy including health.

It is suggested that many studies have been but subtle variants of a major theme which focuses on culture, and fails to address itself to the fundamental issue of race and racism. It is not suggested, however, that all studies have been uncritical of the power relations and dominant social structures which mediate them, or that scholars have remained fixed in their stance, ostrich-like and unaware of the criticism and debate [7,8]. Nor is it suggested that these studies have been <u>intentionally</u> diversionary, fudging the issue. To suggest so would be to misunderstand the nature of institutionalised racism. However, to ignore the criticism and to fail to reflect on the implications for these studies and their relation to policies would amount to collusion with and perpetuation of the racist ideologies which permeate our society and thinking.

Cultural Pluralism and Ethnic Diversity: A Decoy from Racism

The dominant approach of 'race relations/ethnic minority' studies has been within a framework of cultural pluralism and ethnic diversity. The relationship between culturally 'distinct' minorities [9] and majority white society is seen exclusively in terms of culture, apparently autonomous although interacting with other social processes. It is diversity and difference in languages, religions and cultural 'norms' or expectations which prevent effective communication and create misunderstandings between the majority and the 'distinct' minorities. 'Problems' are therefore the result of mismatches between minority and majority cultures which, according to the pluralist view, meet on equal terms. Any imbalances in 'the ethnic relations equation' are therefore attributed to the relative 'weight' of culture on either or both sides [10]. The assumption that both sides of the situation are subject to the <u>same</u> political/economic forces means that tinkering with cultural differences until there are 'equal components' on each side will get the

balance   —   and   therefore   communication and
understanding — right and solve the 'problem'.
   A   major   point   at   issue   is   the   essential
approach   of   the pluralist perspective. Society and
its   ideology   are   unproblematic, the potential for
adequate   reforms being taken for granted.   The only
necessary   ingredient   is   good sound information on
culture   —   the   cause   of the mismatch and problem.
This denies a major political dimension, and culture
itself   becomes   problematic.   Within   the   largely
uncritical   framework,   the   outcome   is to focus on
minority   culture.   It   is   then a small and almost
imperceptible   step   to   locate   the   cause   of   the
mismatch   and   problems in the minorities themselves
and   their culture which is different.   Adherents of
the   cultural   pluralist   school would deny that the
minorities   are   held   responsible for communication
and   cultural   problems   and   difficulties.   Their
argument   may   well   be that multiculturalism is the
only   way   to proceed, promoting understanding on all
sides   of   the   others   cultures and points of view.
None   would   deny   that differences in languages and
ways   of   seeing   the   world   can   prevent effective
communication and generate misunderstandings.
   The   point   at   issue   is   not   the   fact   of
linguistic   or cultural difference, nor the need for
sensitive   understanding,   but   the value judgements
placed   on   that   difference as deviant, alien and
stubborn   —   in   short,   a   problem.   At issue
is   the   central   assumption   of   pluralists, that
different   cultures   meet   on   equal   terms.   This is
the   nub: that   the   'classic'   dominant   ethnic
relations   school mislocates race relations entirely
in   the   sphere   of   culture   outside   the political
arena [11].   Such   an   approach   obscures and denies
the   crucial   historical   and   contemporary   power
relations   of   race   which have created an imbalance
between   certain   'culturally   distinct'   groups.
There   has   been   an essential lack of criticism, in
that   white   'experts'   or a broadly descriptive and
ethnocentric   anthropological tradition have studied
'exotic'   minority cultures, whilst their ability to
provide sound, objective information has rarely been
questioned.   The   relations   of   race   operating
between   the   white   researcher and the black/ethnic
minority   research   object have slipped past largely
ignored and unexamined.
   Black   and   ethnic   minorities are not therefore
merely   numerically   small   groups   of people with a
distinct   culture   attributed with equal importance.

They are seen as inferior and subordinate by the dominant majority, with whom relations are imbued with notions of inferiority, alienness and pathogenesis [12]. To see ethnic relations as a temporarily imbalanced cultural equation, the resolution of which merely requires some tinkering with cultural factors, is to hopelessly miss the point. The relations more closely resemble an immobilised see-saw heavily weighted by the subordinate minorities 'culture'. Balance necessitates not just that they shed some of that weight, but that they also drag themselves up the steep incline to 'integrate' with the unproblematic dominant white majority at the other end. This is the solution implicit in the uncritical pluralist approach, rather than a shift in the fulcrum of power, which would in itself help to redress the balance.

Their perspective also fudges the issues, serving as a powerful decoy. It is not just that it 'lets white society off the hook', but that it categorically excludes the experience of people who feel the same as the rest of the British population: who speak English, eat fish and chips perhaps, drink beer, are possibly nominal Christians but who are black. In short, in failing to address the issue of race, this approach does not address their experience.

Different Cultures: Alien, Deviant and Pathological

One of the most salient features of the emphasis on culture is its inherent and subtle contradiction. Whilst acting as a powerful decoy from racism, it nevertheless reflects its nature, by emphasising difference as alien, deviant, abnormal and pathological [13,14]. Studies which focus on minority culture, but do not take an explicitly anti-racist view, reflect (albeit unintentionally) an ethnocentric view that 'white (English/ Protestant) is right'. Since blame is often implicitly apportioned to minority cultures, so it is a logical extension to see such cultures as deviant and pathological. It is precisely because the research findings of white 'experts', often uncritical of the social relations which structure their field work and analysis, are eagerly awaited by policy makers and professionals alike, that we need to take a closer look at what 'different culture' is often taken to mean.

105

It is around the issue of <u>difference</u> that there is complex and often contradictory discussion. On the one hand descriptions of the particular differences peculiar to each group are an integral part of the culturalist approach, whilst the 'common alienness' is also an issue [15]. Minorities are alien first, and distinct (ethnic) second. To ignore differences is seen by some as an egalitarian approach, treating all people the same, but by others as evidence of race/colour blindness. To recognise difference is to reinforce and emphasise divisive notions of alienness to some, whilst to others it is a prerequisite for a sensitive awareness, and a welcome departure from ethnocentrism.

These cultural differences of 'alien' origin are imbued with perjorative connotations of inferiority within an uncritical view of white society as the 'norm'. The 'generation conflicts' between young Asian girls/women and their parents are somehow seen as being of a different order [16] than the long known 'generation gap' in English society which resulted in the need for agencies such as GALS (Girls Alone in London Service). Rather than generation gaps being universal, their existence within 'Asian' families in Britain is taken to show how inflexible and inappropriate the 'traditional Asian family' is to life in Britain (alien) and the problems it causes for the children (pathological). The matrifocal family in West Indian culture, and the higher number of children who are 'illegitimate' by English standards of the nuclear family, is often cited as a similar instance of culture which in itself causes problems for the mother and children [17,18], and therefore for the welfare services.

Such problems, rooted in different cultures, were clearly 'imported' during the 1950s and 1960s, when immigration from the New Commonwealth and Pakistan was at its height. Those who have 'integrated' (assimilated/become British) are clearly not a problem: it is those who steadfastly refuse to do so. Muslim women who are seen as 'cloistered' or 'imprisoned' in purdah cause 'problems' for services such as the NHS when they attend clinics and neither speak English nor submit to the requirements that they should be examined by a male doctor. All too often one hears the old adage 'when in Rome . . .' a view reflected in the failure of many services to provide interpreters.

The responsibility for communication and 'integration' lies (un)fairly and squarely at the door of the minority which speaks an 'alien' language.

The 'alien' family necessarily becomes the focus of cultural studies, as it plays an important part in the reproduction of culture. There is also the view that the minority family is the subject of interest because it is one of the few remaining bastions of autonomy from white society [19]. The Asian 'arranged' marriage is often the subject of considerable interest: being so 'alien' to the principle of 'free choice', it is difficult to understand how marital problems are avoided in such an enforced situation. Similarly, the extended Asian family with more children and with more generations under one roof (generating conflict) is as deviant but strangely enough as 'strong' as the West Indian family is 'weak' [20].

Clearly ethnic minorities cannot win; and the positive aspects of their life style even by 'British' standards are rarely mentioned. The extended family, for example where it exists in Britain provides support and prevents isolation particularly of elderly people, or of young mothers, that have been lost in the English nuclear family.

THE HISTORY AND IDEOLOGY OF WESTERN MEDICINE

The Emergence of Mechanistic, Scientific Medicine

Contemporary Western medicine is but one particular medical tradition, the methodology and concepts of which are rooted in the mechanistic view of life which gained supremacy in the 19th century. Previously medicine had developed within a tradion of 'vitalism', with its holistic view of life and disease. This approach was manifest in medical practice as an active and responsive dialogue between the sick person and the practitioner. Arguably as important in determining the nature of medical practice were the social and political relations within which it was practised. In the 18th century, the clients were wealthy patrons who paid doctors to observe and cure their symptoms. The doctor's wit and good company, as much as their technical competence and skill, were probably factors deciding the wealthy client's endowment of patronage [21,22].

The mechanistic view of life, won acceptance as positivism became the established philosophy and methodology of natural science in the 19th century. It originated in the Cartesian view of the body as dissociated from the soul, perceived as a mere set of component parts, each with discrete functions, whose workings could be explained on purely mechanistic grounds. Within this view, the fundamental unit of life is the inanimate cell, within and between which biochemical interactions take place. Deviation from these normal processes resulted in disease, which can be precisely and objectively identified [23].

The emergence of the hospital as an institution for dealing with the problem of the ill and dying urban poor changed the entire framework of relations between the practitioner and the sick person [24]. The medical men were released from their dependence on the wealthy elite. As they treated ill people who were poor, the balance of power in the dialogue shifted radically in favour of the doctor. The era of the patron was over.

The emphasis in medical practice changed from the art of subjective empathy and observation of the sick person to the science of objective examination of 'cases' of deviant organic matter, and the classification of specific diseases according to pathology, rather than symptoms. With the decline of patronage, it was possible to innovate in medical practice, particularly within hospital institutions, with the captive population of potential research objects [25]. Medical practitioners now able to retreat behind an array of jargon, tests, procedures and equipment became detached from the sick person. The patient became increasingly alienated from the failing set of mechanisms which were yielded submissively to the medical mechanic for repair. A series of diagnostic tests and procedures had to be endured <u>patiently</u>, rather like a pit stop during a motor racing Grand Prix. The major problem with such 'pit stops' for an ill person is that, although the body is treated as a mere mechanism dissociated from the self and soul, it cannot be taken in for repair, left and collected later. The relationship between doctor and patient therefore has to be of a personal nature, within which the body is treated as separate from the mind and soul. Hence the entry into a contract of submission and yielding involving expropriation of decisions and control over one's health whilst being held morally responsible for the biological deviance [26].

The Implications of the Mechanistic View of Disease for Medical Ideology

The mechanistic view of disease, with its simplistic biological explanations, discrete from the socio-economic environment has several important implications. It paves the way for the depersonalisation of the experience of being ill [27]. It also heralded a view of illness as biological deviance from the normal workings of the body. In locating the major determinants of such deviance in the personal sphere of habits and hygiene, the individual careless enough to become ill was held morally responsible for the misdemeanour. The biological agents of disease were simplistically seen as the cause, which could be avoided by healthy living. The role of such agents as but mediating links in a chain of predisposing and determining socio-economic factors, such as appalling living and working conditions, was not acknowledged.

The hegemony of the view has been maintained, despite well-documented evidence that the decline in infectious diseases such as tuberculosis began as living conditions improved and overcrowding decreased. Immunisation was introduced at a late stage, when the incidence rate was already dramatically reduced [28]. Sharp social class, gradients in the incidence of preventable illness have been much publicised [29], including studies showing strong links between unemployment and ill-health [30]. The strong association of much of this illness with social deprivation has not led to the success of a public health movement campaigning vigorously for the abolition of such pathogenic social conditions. The individualistic victim and culture-blaming ideology of medicine has retained its supremacy. It is not surprising, therefore, that the major thrust of the majority of preventive medicine has been on education of the ignorant into health habits. The feasibility of such measures within poor, damp, living conditions; or in a situation of rising unemployment is rarely considered.

There is a second implication of the mechanistic view for medical practice. Unifactoral explanations of the biological nature and cause of disease demand unifactoral solutions, such as pharmaceutical and scientific medical treatment. Whilst responsiblilty for health and disease is attributed to the culture and habits of the person careless enough to become ill, the power and control over treatment and cure is expropriated [31]. This is the preserve and jealously guarded domain of the highly trained professionals, admission to whose elite ranks is rigidly controlled. Whilst the number of women entering the medical and scientific research professions is increasing, those involved in professional practice, research or policy-making are still predominantly white middle-class men.

Subtle contradictions are now emerging. The onus for ill-health is placed on the individual, yet health education to correct 'unhealthy' behaviour is underfinanced and of low status within medical circles. Professional control has not only secured glamour, status and therefore finance for technocratic medicine, but it has also attained unquestioned control over treatment. It is as if, having wilfully failed to heed the health education, the ill person then pays the price in depersonalised treatment over which they have no effective control [32].

THE ARTICULATION OF ETHNIC RELATIONS SOCIOLOGY AND MEDICAL IDEOLOGIES IN ETHNIC MINORITY HEALTH STUDIES AND POLICIES

Common Themes Focusing on Culture

There are conceptual themes which are common to the dominant schools of thought in ethnic relations and medicine, though one must reiterate that these are generalisations which do not apply to all researchers or practitioners. In both fields there is an emphasis on 'healthy' norms, deviations from which are pathological or pathogenic. By definition, there is a strong element of selection in the approved norms of behaviour such as white, middle-class family life, to which the majority of people in Britain probably do not conform. Whilst eating fish and chips and other fatty foods is emphasised as being associated with heart disease, there are not similar exhortations to prevent stress in the executive life style which is similarly associated. These points are intended to be far from flippant or over-simplistic. Clearly there are aspects of everyone's life which contribute to health and/or to ill health. The major point at issue in both debates is the value judgement and relative 'weight' attributed to an individual's habits and culture compared with other socio-economic and political structural factors.

The Politics of Ethnic Minority Health Issues

There are other related dimensions to the study and interpretations of ethnic minorities' health issues. Until recently, the focus on cultural distinctiveness or racial difference as an explanatory factor per se has led to some misleading and simplistic conclusions and definitions of 'problems'. Over-generalisations abound, and the influence of social factors such as occupational class, unemployment and housing conditions are often denied in simplistic analyses which reduce such complex social phenomena to grossly overgeneralised stereotyped racial and ethnic categories. Such interpretations neglect the subtle and crucial effects of racism and racial discrimination.

A recent paper Ethnic Differences in Certified Sickness Absence [33] acknowledged that minority ethnic groups might live in difficult social circumstances as a result of racism, but these were dismissed as a major influence on absence from work. This is a notoriously grey area for all workers, but the authors appear uninformed of relevant research. Their conclusions are cast in terms of 'Asian' households and there is a cavalier disregard of basic data on wage levels of the minority groups and the numbers of dependents.

Gross assumptions were made that the Asian employees

. . . . . . tend to live in larger, more closely knit family units in which there will be several wage earners in one house. The financial consequences of absence from work may be less acute so that there is less pressing need to continue to work when in a state of minor ill health . . . . [34]

Besides the gross generalisation that all 'Asian' employees live in larger households, the possibility that there may be fewer wage earners per members of the household is neither entertained nor empirically refuted. Furthermore, in a context of high unemployment and competition for jobs, such conclusions serve, unwittingly perhaps, to bolster discrimination in employment practices already documented [35]. Similar instances of crude analyses reduced to ethnicity occur in early literature on perinatal health [36] in which, 'Asian' births are compared with 'British' births, and a significantly higher perinatal mortality rate is identified amongst 'Asian' babies. There is an offensive implication that the 'Asians' are not 'British' which of course the majority are. Although the importance of social class as a factor in perinatal health was acknowledged in the paper, its 'effects' in terms of accounting for the apparent difference between ethnic groups was not explicit.

More recent papers have incorporated standardisations and controls for factors such as social class [37,38]. One paper goes further to examine other factors known to be important such as the expertise of those given antenatal care. It was found that "Asian patients (in Leicestershire) have a larger proportion of general practitioners who are not on the obstetric list than non-Asian patients" [39]

The Role of Research in Informing Policy and Practice

Is such a sophisticated analysis enough to allay fears of over-simplistic interpretations which are racist in their definition of minority cultures as deviant and pathogenic? Unfortunately not, for there it remains to consider the barbed issue of the relation of research to policy and practice.

Two of the papers already cited also quote attendance figures at antenatal clinics [40]. In Bradford, it was found that between 1975-78 approximately 60% of "Asian women received less than 4 months supervised antenatal care, compared with 20% of white European women" [41]. Similarly, the study in Leicester found that "at 16 weeks gestation 64% of Asians compared with 80% of non-Asians are enrolled into systematic care" [42].

These findings are apparently harmless enough, but to what use is it put? Does one take the easier route, and define Asian women as a problem because they do not avail themselves of the services provided? Or does one take the alarming disparity as a starting point to find out why the services are not used. Is it because they are not well publicised, or because they are inaccessible?

As discussed in chapter 1, access may have geographical, social or religious dimensions. Services may be underused because they are physically difficult to reach by public transport. Local community clinics may be within easier reach for young mothers with several young children than new district hospitals built on the periphery of towns and cities. If staff are over-professional in their attitudes, overtly racist or intangibly unhelpful, people may find the services socially

112

inaccessible. For many women, the choice of consulting a female doctor influences the accessibility of services, and has led to the growth of well-women's centres, and feminist psychotherapy.

The many factors influencing accessibility must be considered in the interpretation of data on service use. The way the implications are defined and tackled depends very much on how the service and its consumers are perceived. To some, any patient who does not conform to the universal uniform services is a problem. Others who endorse the view that the service is there for the patient, would take positive action to discover whether the service was unacceptable.

But still the pitfalls of lapsing into an essentially cultural view persist. Does one look for unacceptability in terms of specific religious or other traditions which are not catered for (creating problems) or should one also look at direct and indirect racism which might affect the way in which those traditions are viewed, even if apparently catered for?

CONCLUSIONS: THE AGENDA FOR RESEARCH

Of necessity, this has been a brief and generalised review of the major themes which have permeated studies of ethnic minority health. What is to be made of this complex debate? Clearly it has implications for future research, not least because findings do, and have, shape(d) public policy and professional practice. A major consideration is therefore whether the research findings facilitate and enable the struggle of minorities against oppressive structures and improve their access to health; or whether the findings serve to continue the over-emphasis on culture and the need for superficial tinkering to make 'communication' more effective. A major criticism which must be heeded is that cultural pluralist studies, by locating solution within the arena of controlled policy and reform, actively remove them from the arena of power relations and radical changes.

The direction for future research is found in the major criticism for policy-oriented research, that the liaison has been positive and uncritical. Policy and practice have been the raison d'etre of research, rather than the objects under scrutiny. Instead of concluding that race relations research should not be conducted, such criticism should lead to a re-orientation of the focus of such research: whether the 'distinctiveness' of people is viewed within a positive, anti-racist perspective, which categorically rejects notions of alienness, inferiority and deviance. From this perspective difference is not in itself a <u>problem</u>: it is a fact and is not related to an established (white) 'norm'. To focus on difference without the basis of an analysis of power relations of race, as has been seen, is to set one's self on the slippery slope to uncritical pluralism and definitions of ethnic people and their cultures and the <u>problem</u>.

It is imperative that 'cultural studies' do not result in more ethnic minority labels and categories which detract from and minimise the political dimension of their situation. Those who are white 'professional' researchers, are in an attributed position of power in their relations with black people and ethnic minorities with whom they may wish to work. This clearly has implications for what, and whom they study, and whether information-laden research should be done at all. They have to be aware that research which has been conducted with the 'best' of intentions can and has been used in ways detrimental to the interests of those whose experience it was intended to improve. It is not an easy issue. An explicit recognition that white society, its policies and practice is a fundamental determinant of black people's experience and access to health must necessarily have implications for the relations between researcher and researched, and for the agenda and orientation of that research.

REFERENCES

1. Jenkins, R. (1971) <u>The Production of Knowledge at the Institute of Race Relations</u>, Independent Labour Party Publications
2. Mullard, C. (1973) <u>Black Britain</u>, Allen and Unwin, London
3. Sivanandan, A (1976) Race, class and the state, <u>Race and Class</u>, Vol. 17, pp. 347-368
4. Smith, D.J. (1976) The facts of racial disadvantage, Vol. XLII Broadsheet No. 560, Political and Economic Planning, London

5. Joint Tuberculosis Committee of the British Thoracic Society (1982) Control and prevention of tuberculosis: a code of practice, British Medical Journal, Vol. 287, pp. 1118-1121
6. Ben-Tovim, G. and Gabriel, J. (1982) The sociology of race- time to change course, in A. Ohri, B. Manning and P. Curno (eds) Community Work and Racism, Routledge Kegan Paul, London
7. Khan, V. (1979) Migration and social stress, in V. Khan (ed) Minority Families in Britain, Macmillan
8. Khan, V. (1982) The role of the culture of dominance in structuring the experience of ethnic minorities, in C. Husband (ed) Race in Britain, Hutchinson, London
9. Ben-Tovim, G. and Gabriel, J. (1982) op. cit.
10. Lawrence, E. (1982) In the abundance of water the fool is thirsty, The Empire Strikes Back, Centre for Contemporary Cultural Studies, Hutchinson
11. Ibid.
12. Ibid.
13. Ibid.
14. Parmer, P (1981) Young Asian women: a critique of the pathological approach, Multiracial Education, Vol. 9, pp. 19-29
15. Lawrence, E. (1982) op. cit.
16. Parmer, P. (1981) op. cit.
17. Lawrence, E. (1982) op. cit.
18. Palmer, P. (1981) op. cit.
19. Lawrence, E. (1981) White sociology, black struggle, Multiracial Education, Vol. 9, pp. 3 -17
20. Ibid.
21. Jewson, N. (1976) The disappearance of the sick man from medical cosmology 1778-1870, Sociology, Vol. 10, pp. 225-244
22. Jewson, N. (1974) Medical knowledge and the patronage system in eighteenth century England, Sociology, Vol. 8, pp. 369-385
23. Ibid.
24. Waddington, I. (1973) The role of the hospital in the development of modern medicine: a sociological analysis, Sociology, Vol. 7, pp. 211-224
25. Ibid.

26. Figlio, K. (1971) The historiography of scientific medicine: an invitation to the human sciences, Comparative Studies in Society and History, Vol. 19, pp. 265
27. Illich, I. (1975) Medical Nemesis, Penguin, Harmondsworth
28. McKeown, T. and Record, R.G. (1974) Reasons for the decline in mortality in England and Wales during the nineteenth century, in M.W. Flinn. and T.C. Smart (eds) Essays in Social History, Clarendon Press, Oxford, pp.
29. Townsend, P. and Davidson, N. (1982) Inequalities in Health, Penguin, Harmondsworth
30. Colledge, M. (1982) Unemployment and Health, North Tyneside Community Health Council
31. Illich, I. (1975) op. cit.
32. Ibid.
33. Barker, C.C. and Pocock, S.J. (1983) Ethnic differences in certified sickness absence, British Journal of Industrial Medicine, Vol. 39, pp. 277-282
34. Ibid, pp. 281
35. Allen, S. and Smith C.R. (1975) Minority group experience: the transition from education to work, in P. Brannen (ed) Entering the World of Work: Some Sociological Perspectives, H.M.S.O, London
36. Lumb, K.M., Congden, P.J. AND Lealman, G.T. (1981) A comparative review of Asian and British born maternity patients in Bradford 1974-1978, Journal Epidemiology and Community Health, Vol.35, pp. 106-109
37. Clarke, M. and Clayton, D.G. (1983) Quality of obstetric care provided for Asian immigrants in Leicestershire, British Medical Journal, Vol. 286, pp. 621-3
38. Terry, P.B., Condie, R.G. and Settatree, R.S. (1981) Analysis of ethnic differences in perinatal statistics, British Medical Journal, Vol. 281, pp. 1307-8
39. Clarke, M.and Clayton, D.G. op. cit.
40. Lumb, K. et al (1981) op. cit.
41. Clarke, M. and Clayton D.G. (1983) op. cit.
42. Lumb, K. et al (1981) op. cit.

Chapter 5

BLACK PEOPLE's HEALTH: A DIFFERENT APPROACH

Jenny Donovan

INTRODUCTION

Evidence about the health of black people in Britain
is 'patchy and somewhat inconclusive' according to
the Black Report Inequalities in Health [1,2],
supposedly the most detailed analysis of health in
Britain to date. The research which has been done
has tended to concentrate on a few topics and ethnic
groups at the expense of others, and has largely
ignored the views of the black population. Mostly,
researchers have looked at conditions which they
believe affect specific ethnic groups, such as
sickle-cell anaemia in people of Afro-Caribbean
descent, and rickets in people of Asian descent; or
on topics of special interest to themselves, such as
schizophrenia, tuberculosis and venereal disease.
On the whole, the approach employed has been to
isolate black individuals and groups, to discuss
them as 'problems', and then to go on to suggest
solutions that are couched entirely in terms of
individuals themselves having to change their ways
of life so that they will conform to the desired
norm of the white majority [3].
    Implicit in this work, and sometimes explicit,
is the blaming of individuals or their cultures for
ill-health. Hence people of Asian descent have
been criticised for having diets which are seen to
be a major cause of rickets and low
birthweights [4,5]; and Afro-Caribbean family
structures have been implicated in causing high
child accident rates and in the development of
schizophrenia [6,7]. At best, this sort of research
is insensitive; at worst it shows a complete
ignorance of non-European cultures and ways of life
as Pearson has eminently demonstrated (chapter
four).
    The tendency for researchers to fall into the
trap of 'blaming the victim' is particularly obvious
in the case of rickets and mental health. Although

117

researchers agree that "it seems that vitamin D deficiency is the major factor leading to rickets and osteomalacia among Indian and Pakistani immigrants to Britain" [8]; they disagree over the precise causes of the affliction and over particular solutions.   It is considered that a deficiency of vitamin D may be caused by any of the following: the misuse or lack of adequate supplements, the possible inhibition of the absorption of the vitamin by phytate in chapattis (a popular Asian food made with wholemeal flour), a lack of sunshine, and dietary deficiencies.   In recent years, the last two have received the most attention.

It is claimed, for example, that the average Asian diet does not provide adequate quantities of vitamin D, because it tends not to contain foods naturally rich in the vitamin, such as oily fish, and because many people choose to use butter for frying food rather than fortified margarine [9,10]. For some researchers, the solution is clear: "the long term answer to Asian rickets probably lies in health education and a change towards the Western diet and life-style" [11].   For others, such a solution is inappropriate, and a more suitable proposal is the fortification of a popular food, such as chapattis because, as they point out, rickets was only eradicated among the white poor when margarine was fortified [12].

A lack of sunshine is now thought to be the most important cause of vitamin D deficiency because the action of ultra-violet light on the skin stimulates the production of large quantities of the vitamin [13].   Arneil and Crosbie [14] suggest that rickets occurs in Asians because "dusky skin requires more ultra-violet radiation than white skin", but their evidence is sparse and they fail to explain why people of Afro-Caribbean descent do not exhibit such high rates of rickets as Asians. Other writers suggest that Asian, and particularly Muslim culture is to blame, because it may prevent women from exposing their skin to sunlight [15]. These authors ignore the possibility that people might not want to sunbathe, or that they may live in areas without parks and gardens, or where racist attacks or fear force people to stay inside.

The policy of the Department of Health and Social Security (DHSS) [16] has been to rely for now on the use of supplements, to encourage Asians to spend more time outside, and to advocate that they should westernise their diets.   This policy has been severely criticised because it assumes that the

Western way is right, and the Asian diets and
cultural/religious practices are to blame for the
incidence of rickets. It is but a short step to
suggest that Asians themselves are to blame for the
condition, and thereby deflect attention away from
the real causes of the complaint: inadequate and
poor housing in run-down, sometimes hostile inner-
city areas, and the lack of a fortified popular
food.
     In the field of mental health, research has
been undertaken to try to understand migrant
behaviour and to explain the effects of migration on
mental health. On the whole, it is suggested that
moving from a poor rural area or city in the Third
World to a large British city is a stressful
experience, and that when this is compounded by
'culture shock' and racial discrimination, high
rates of mental illness are only to be
expected [17,18]. A contradiction arises, however,
when one looks at studies of actual use of
psychiatric services, where it appears that black
people do not use these as much as white people do.
Asians in particular use the services rarely. For
people of Afro-Caribbean descent, their rates for
depressive illnesses are very low, but for
schizophrenia and paranoia, they are very much
higher than other groups [19,20]. In addition, by no
means all ethnic group members are now migrants.
     These contradictions are explained away by
writers by suggesting that there may be a fault in
the services, or that a large proportion of real
illness must be concealed by families, or that
ethnic groups must provide sufficient non-
professional treatment to prevent the mentally ill
from turning to the services. It has also been
suggested that differences in the presentation of
symptoms by different groups, and the different
expectations of doctors may be of importance [21].
Before this was suggested, it was assumed that the
culture of West Indians in particular caused
schizophrenia, just as it was thought that Asian
diets were responsible for rickets. An analysis of
the numbers diagnosed as schizophrenic and the
reasons for their diagnosis has revealed, however, a
basic ethnocentricity in doctors' training and there
is also evidence to suggest that differential
treatment may occur áccording to race [22].
     In the case of mental illness as well as
rickets, then, researchers have tended to place the
blame for the conditions on the culture of members
of ethnic minority groups. This ethnocentric

short-sightedness   is   now   being   exposed and
denounced,   but   the   influence   of past research is
pervasive   and   there   is   still   a   tendency to
concentrate   on the 'unusual' illnesses and diseases
which   affect   relatively few black people [23]. The
critiques   of   the   traditional sort of research are
few.   The   paper   by   Webb [24]   stands   out here,
because it is an analysis of health worries reported
by   black   people   to   a   radio   programme, and
consequently avoids 'exotic' conditions.   Similarly
the   pamphlet by Brent Community Health Council [25]
stands   out because it represents an attempt to link
black   people's   health   to   political   factors,
including   racism.   This   chapter   represents an
attempt to combine these two alternative approaches:
the   disassociation   of   'exotic'   diseases and
cultures   as   a   predisposing   variable,   with the
enhancement of the political dimension in which such
studies must be placed.

HISTORY OF IMMIGRATION

It   is   not the purpose here to look in depth at the
history   of   immigration   and   and   settlement in
Britain   [26],   but   it   is   essential   that the
historical   background is not ignored.   Black people
have lived in Britain since the time of Elizabeth I,
but   it   has been only since the end of World War II
that   they   have   settled   in larger numbers.   First
West Indians and later Southern Asians were drawn to
Britain   in   the late 1950s and 1960s to take up job
opportunities   that   were   perceived   to exist [27].
These   jobs   were   generally   poorly   paid, with bad
working   conditions,   long hours and few promotional
prospects.   Since the jobs were largely to be found
in   or   close   to   the   decaying inner city areas of
Britain's larger cities, the immigrants were obliged
to   find accommodation nearby, often renting, buying
or   getting   mortgages   on   run down properties with
poor facilities and little space [28,29].
        Since   the   curtailing   of   immigration   by the
Commonwealth   Immigrants   Acts of 1962 and 1968, the
Immigration   Act of 1971, and the Nationality Act of
1981,   the position of black people has changed very
little.   As   the   PEP   Reports   have shown [30,31],
black people still live in some of the worst quality
housing,   private   and   council;   black workers are

still over-represented in the manufacturing or low-
grade service sectors, working long hours or shifts
for lower than average pay, and few have gained
promotion.
    The effects of work on health are known to be
enormous   [32,33],   but there have been few attempts
to link the 'race relations' research with that
concerning health. Although some authors admit that
poverty and poor housing may be responsible for some
diseases such as tuberculosis, few pay any attention
to the action of racial discrimination on health.
The   documentary   evidence   of   the disadvantage
suffered by black people is, however well known [34-
38] and the effects of this disadvantage cannot be
anything but enormous.

BLACK PEOPLE SPEAK OUT ABOUT THEIR HEALTH

Black studies and 'race relations' research have not
only failed to tackle major issues of importance,
but they have also neglected to ask black people
what they think and feel about their own lives and
health.   Such omissions are not unexpected when
most of the work done in the field has had a
positivistic approach, based either upon medical
statistics or conventional social survey.
    The author is still undertaking research, the
aim of which is to understand the perceptions and
experiences of health and the health services of a
group of black people living in London.   The
emphasis is on the understanding of how and why
people act or do not act when their health is
threatened, and the study is set in the context of
their own lives and the contrasting and sometimes
contradictory needs and wants they may feel.   The
focus throughout is on the individual, and her/his
interpretation of her/his life is the primary
concern. The work focuses on case-studies, examined
in detail, using loosely structured interviews which
encourage people to tell stories about their
experiences. This approach emphasises the wholeness
and uniqueness of each individual, and allows the
free expression of views and opinions in context.
    Thirty people were contacted and interviewed
between October 1982 and October 1983. Of these,
twenty-four are women, of whom eight were born in
the West Indies, seven in India, six in Pakistan,
two in Ghana and one in Kenya. Five of the women
of Afro-Caribbean descent were first contacted via
the workplace of a fellow (part-time) research

student,   and   they in turn introduced me to six men
and   two more women.   The other three women of Afro-
Caribbean   descent   were   contacted   separately.   Of
the six men, three were born in the West Indies, and
three   in   Britain.   The   fourteen   women   of Asian
descent   form   part   of   a   small   community in East
London,   and   all   attend   the   same   local club.   A
social   worker   introduced   the author to one of the
women   (Naseem),   and   she   was willing to act as an
interpreter and to contact the other women.

     All   the   subjects   were   seen   at   least once.
For   the   first meeting, a loosely arranged schedule
of   questions was used which encouraged the subjects
to   talk   about   health   and   illness   from their
childhood   to   the   present,   and   the   order of the
material   was   largely dependent on what they wanted
to   discuss.   All the interviews were tape-recorded,
and   lasted   between   one hour, and three-and-three-
quarter hours.   They   were   fully transcribed.   The
material   appeared   to   fall   into   a   number of
interlinked   sections,   concerned   respectively with
childhood,   remedies, other people's health, general
practitioners   (GPs),   hospitals,   private medicine,
racism,   food,   religion,   work, the government, the
police,   housing,   education   and the future.   After
close   scrutiny of the material, it was decided that
a   return to some of the subjects would be useful to
pursue   further some of the things only touched upon
initially, this time using a more focused approach.

     It   is   not   possible   here   to give a detailed
account   of the wealth of the material gathered, and
so   the   discussion will begin with some information
about the subjects, goes on to consider some general
findings   about   health   and   illness, and concludes
with   a   few   observations   on   the relevance of the
findings [39].

SUBJECTS

The   ten   women   of   Afro-Caribbean descent are aged
between   24   and 58 years, and all were born outside
the   UK.   Eight   came   to   Britain   to   join their
families   or   husbands and two to work on the advice
of   relatives.   At   the   time of the first contact,
eight   of   the   women   were working full-time: (Ivy,
Delores,   Millie,   Ruby,   Judy,   Donna,   Jean and
Martha);   the two others (Emily and Louise) were too
ill   to   work.   Emily   and Louise have no children,
the   others   have   had between one and six.   The six
men   of   Afro-Caribbean   descent are aged between 21

and 57 years. One came to Britain after being
recruited by British Rail; two came to join their
parents, and the other three were born in Britain.
At the time of first contact, all were working full-
time and two were working shifts: Joe and Carlton,
who was doing permanent nights. Only Joe was
married (to Jean), and they have five children –
three of whom were interviewed (Earl, Danny and
Paul). Earl lives with his girlfriend and two
children; Leroy had moved out with his girlfriend
and child by the time of the last interview; and
the other men are single and childless.

The fourteen women of Asian descent are aged
between 19 and 60ish (the oldest woman was unsure of
her age), and all were born outside the UK. At the
time of first contact, three of the women were doing
some paid work: Taresh, Geeta and Shobha. Only
Rani and Farida have no children; the others have
had between two and eight. The majority of the
interviews were conducted in Urdu by Naseem,
although Punjabi and Hindi were also used.
Tasneem, Sufiya, Dalee and Shobha were able to
answer some questions in English, and Naseem's
interview was conducted entirely in English.

HEALTH AND ILLNESS

Not surprisingly, all the women agree that good
health is extremely important to them. The older
women feel that they need good health to be able to
enjoy their lives and to get through all their
tasks; whereas for the younger women with children,
the over-riding need is to be healthy enough to look
after their children. For the men, good health is
more important for their work and so that they can
enjoy themselves. Staying healthy, however, is
generally seen to be a matter of chance or fate, or,
for the religious people, a matter of God's will.
This fatalism was followed up in the second round of
interviews, and the women in particular emphasise
the inevitability of ill-health and their
powerlessness to do anything about it: "Everyone
gets something . . . Whatever you are destined to
get, you will get" (Delores); "You can get ill, any
time of your life. You can never expect that you
will always be healthy" (Naseem); "We can just
take care, but it depends on God. You can still

get ill, any time" (Rani). For the men, staying in
good health is more a matter of being fit enough
to overcome any ill-health: "I usually keep myself
very, very fit, so that if anything comes to
me, I'm strong enough not to take any notice of it"
(Carlton); "if you get an illness, your natural
body resistance will get rid of it" (Paul).

Those seen more than once were asked to talk
about the meaning of an 'illness', and those of
Afro-Caribbean descent were also asked to explain
the difference, if any, between an illness and a
disease. (This was not possible for the Asian women
because there is only one word which covers the
whole concept of ill-health: 'beemaar'). For the
women, to be unwell is "a feelin', somethin' out of
the ordinary" (Delores); or "tiredness. You feel
tired, don't feel like doing any work" (Naseem).
For the men it is much more of an interference:
"anything that keeps me off work for a period of two
or three days" (Earl): "something that stop me from
doin' what I am able to do, which puts me down,
makes me feel sick, feel weak" (Carlton). On the
whole, the Afro-Caribbean women believe that a
disease is much more serious than an illness. Emily
says, for example, "an illness can go, but a disease
is something that you can't cure".

The origins of ill-health are not a great
concern of the people interviewed. For most, ill-
health is accepted for what it is, and its origins
are not as important as its effects. There are
some guesses at causes, however. Several women
mention, for example, that worries can cause
illnesses, or at least run the body down so that it
is more susceptible to ill-health. Delores, Ruby,
Martha and Ivy are particularly concerned about
this, and they make direct links between the
stresses and problems in their lives (including such
things as racism, difficulties within the family or
at work), and various illnesses which they suffer,
such as hypertension (Ivy); high blood pressure and
sugar diabetes (Ruby); high blood pressure
(Delores); and nervous breakdown (Martha).
Tasneem, Reena and Rajinda also feel that there is a
direct link between family worries and ill-health.
For Reena, there are worries about her children's
futures; for Rajinda it is the memories of her
husband and daughter, both of whom died in tragic

124

circumstances;   and   for   Tasneem, it is worries she
believes   she brings on herself by wondering what is
happening to her family and friends in Pakistan.

    Joe   was   the only man to agree that illness was
caused   by   worries.   The others feel that illnesses
'just   happen'.   As Earl says: "(an illness) could
affect one person, and sort of totally miss another.
It's   a   question   of   fate   - who's lucky and who
isn't".   The   men   do,   however, believe that some
illnesses   and   diseases have external causes.   Like
the majority of the women, they believe that 'germs'
can   cause illnesses or diseases, and these are seen
as invading organisms which can be caught from other
people (Emily,   Rani,   Tasneem and Carlton), or get
under   the   skin   (Delores) or are just 'in the air'
(Leroy   and   Earl).   Colds   and coughs are the most
commonly   mentioned   illnesses   caused   by   germs.
Almost   everyone   also   mentions   the body's natural
defences against germs, whether these be white blood
cells   (Emily),   or just 'natural resistance', which
can be affected by the strength of a person.

    Much   time   during   the   interview   was spent
talking   about   each   person's medical history.   No-
one   claimed   to   have   perfect   health at the first
meeting although Jean, Martha, Farh   and   Farida
thought   they were close to this.   The most commonly
mentioned   complaints   overall   were   accidents and
depression, closely followed by colds, headaches and
gynaecological stories, but there were also tales of
great   strength   and resourcefulness in dealing with
some very difficult complaints.

WORK

The   majority   of   people who work believe that this
can   affect   their   health.   Only three of the Asian
women   do   any   paid   work, and Taresh in particular
finds   it   hard: "I   get pains in the eyes and the
muscles   in the shoulders because I have to bend for
long   periods   over   the   machine".   The   pay they
receive   is very poor - sometimes they can earn only
£5   after   working all day, but Geeta and Shobba say
that   despite   this   they   prefer to work because it
helps   to   pass   the   time,   and stops them thinking
about   their   families abroad.   Several of the other
Asian women say they would also like to work to pass
the time, but they are unable to find any.

    For   the people of Afro-Caribbean descent, work
is   a   very   important force in their lives.   All of
them   were   working at the time of the first contact

although by the final contact, Carlton had been made
redundant.   He feels that unemployment damages his
health: "I lost a lot of weight . . . it got to my
mind.   It was really gettin' serious for me."
     Most of the men have dangerous jobs, but they
like their work and do not always mind the risks to
their health.   It is clear that these risks exist:
Leroy has had several absences due to accidents (he
is a scaffolder);   Paul and Earl complain that they
get headaches and nausea from flourescent lights;
Danny worries about getting silicosis from grinders
and being hit by flying metal, but adds that as he
works for a small firm of toolmakers, they have to
take risks to complete orders.   Joe complains about
his irregular shifts which exacerbate his ulcer, and
he worries about the effects of working with
asbestos and other fumes;   and Carlton speaks in the
first interview of the difficulties of working
permanent night shifts and of the chemicals he is
forced to handle that have already scarred one of
his workmates.
     Despite all these risks, the men would all
prefer to have their jobs than to be out of work.
The importance of work to the men in particular can
be seen throughout their interviews, when almost all
of their comments about health and illness refer to
work in some way.
     Five of the women of Afro-Caribbean descent
work as care assistants in an old people's home
(Ivy, Delores, Millie, Ruby, and Judy) and they all
believe the work or the working conditions can have
severe effects on their health.   Judy and Delores
tell of eye infections they have picked up from the
urine of the residents and they and Millie and Ruby
are afraid of what else they might catch from the
old people: "The work we doin' affect you - make
you sick.   The residents you're lookin' after, it
make you sick" (Ruby);   "there's people at work and
they're really smelly, like the ones that suffer
from cancer and Parkinson's . . . Sometimes you can
feel it breathin' down you" (Judy);   "Everythin' you
washin' is terrible smellin'.   Even though there is
no infection there, you can still get something,
'cause is so many old people and all have different
diseases" (Millie).   Ivy and Delores have both had
time off work after accidents at work: Ivy after
dislocating her knee in a fall;   Delores after
straining her back lifting one of the residents, and
damaging her wrist after a fall.   They all talk at
length of the exhaustion they feel after the shifts,

yet Millie also has another night cleaning job because she cannot manage to look after her own and her sister's children on the one low wage.

RACISM

Almost all of the subjects acknowledge the existence of racism, based either on their own or other people's experiences.   Many of the women of Asian descent do not go very far from their homes on their own, and some know very little English, but they all believe that racial abuse and attacks do occur. Naseem is the most aware of verbal racial abuse because she speaks and understands English fully, and she says it does affect and depress her.   Syeda and Tasneem report incidents of white youths throwing things at them and hurling abuse, and Tasneem feels that other white people, "May be they have a certain grudge about us, but they don't show it so much.   They keep it in their heart, whereas the teenagers, they can't hide it."   Naseem and Reena recall that their husbands have faced prejudice at work, and Shobha has particularly strong beliefs because her son has been beaten up at school by white youths: "Mrs Thatcher says immigrants will swamp the country.   The way she talks makes people think we are not good people . . . She keeps being prejudiced, saying immigrants are spoiling the country, making it dirty. All the things we do for the country and she doesn't take any notice of the work she gets from us."
    The area in which the Asian women live is near the school made the centre of media attention early in 1984 for racial attacks on pupils and the arrest of eight Asian youths who fought with plain clothes policemen whom they thought were racists.   The eight youths are known as the 'Newham Eight', and their plight was followed closely by the women, particularly Naseem.   The threats of verbal and physical violence depress and offend the women, but they feel powerless to stop it: "We know these things happen here, and we just have to live with them" (Taresh).
    The women of Afro-Caribbean descent try not to let racism get them down, but it obviously does. For the five who work in the old people's home, the issue is particularly important because they have a racist superior who is intent on getting black people out of the home.   They say she has tried to segregate the workers, with the blacks downstairs

dealing with the hardest cases and the whites upstairs, but Ruby and Delores in particular fought against the policy by reporting it to the Commission for Racial Equality. All five of the women speak of incidents involving this woman, but Ruby and Delores seem most affected. Ruby makes explicit the links between the racism at work and her health, believing that the pressure put on her by the supervisor, combined with the stress of the police arresting her son for 'Sus', caused her sugar diabetes and high blood pressure.

Racism is not confined to the work place alone: "It is there, you can feel it all the time, everywhere. You know you are black" (Ivy). Martha, Donna and Delores speak at great length about racism and its effects with an anger and passion not really expressed elsewhere in the interviews. They, like Shobha, above, have an acute political awareness of the issues and react angrily to media and political party propaganda. One of the effects of racism that they all speak about is the feeling that they are not a part of British society, even though some of them have lived here for more than twenty years. Several still hope to return to the islands, especially Ruby, Delores, Louise and Donna; and they are deeply concerned about their children's futures. Martha, Emily, Delores and Ivy propound the view that people should be treated as "people, not colour" (Martha), and they all believe in equality and fairness. Only one of all the women made a racist comment: Rajinda, who says, "the West Indians are worse with us, worse than the whites, especially in hospitals."

The men of Afro-Caribbean descent speak about racism in their private lives and attempts to get jobs. It bothers them, but, like the women, they try to ignore it and to get on with life. Leroy, Paul, Earl and Carlton all mention occasions when they feel sure that they have been refused employment or promotion because they are black; and Leroy and Earl recall incidents in which they were set upon, verbally and physically, by white youths. Joe is more reticent about racism, claiming that "it's more of a class distinction than the colour . . . the colour is only an excuse . . . it's a matter of envy". All of the men are opposed to racial discrimination, and as Carlton says, "This body, it's jus' the outside of my inside. I jus' lookin' through this skin. What matters is inside."

None   of   the   men   believes   that   they have
received   poor   treatment   under   the   NHS because of
their   colour,   but   a   few   of   the   women do.   The
majority   of the women said initially that they were
happy with their treatment in hospitals, but as they
went   on   to   tell   stories   about   their actual
experiences,   it was apparent that some had had very
poor   treatment   and   that   others   had   been badly
neglected.
Some   of   the   women of Asian descent said that
they   found it very difficult to know what to expect
of   doctors   and   nurses   in   hospital, and what, in
turn,   was   expected of them.   Most of those who had
been   in   hospital recalled that they had often been
left   alone   for   long   periods, and Naseem, Taresh,
Sufiya   and Rajinda remember clearly being told that
they   were making too much noise, too much fuss, and
were   pretending   to   be   ill.   Several other women
seem   to have been made unnecessarily over-conscious
of   the   costs   of the treatment they have received,
and   Sufiya, for example, was made to feel extremely
guilty   for   her   son's   expensive   thalassaemia
treatment.   Tasneem mentions that when doctors were
unable   to   diagnose   what   was wrong with her, they
suggested   that the cause was probably the result of
her   unhappy marriage.   In fact, she had TB, and her
marriage   was   perfectly happy.   At a meeting of the
women to discuss the NHS, several said that they had
been   transferred   to private treatment by their GPs
without   their agreement, and consequently forced to
pay   for   consultation   and prescriptions which they
were entitled to have free under the NHS.
Some   of   the   women of Afro-Caribbean descent
were   more   willing   to   specify occasions when they
thought   they had received poor treatment because of
their   colour.   Millie,   for   example, tells of the
hospital   which fitted her with a contraceptive coil
immediately   after   the birth of her third child who
was   suffering   from   sickle-cell anaemia.   She says
that   this   occurred   without   her   knowledge and
permission,   and   that it was unnecessary because in
her   culture,   women   do not sleep with a man for at
least   three   months   after the birth.   The story is
particularly   harrowing   because   of   the   repeated
fitting of coils against her will, the terrible pain
she   suffered   as   a   result   of   these   coils, the
incidents   with   doctors   who   told her that she was
hysterical   and imagining the pain, and her eventual
need   to   have   a hysterectomy.   She makes the links
between   the   contraceptive   coil   and   the fibroids
which   necessitated   the   hysterectomy   clearly, and

recounts that the doctor who treated her badly did
so "because he doesn't like blacks" (Millie) and,
because she is unmarried, and uses the title Miss
rather than Mrs. Judy also mentions an experience
with a young hospital doctor who refused to treat a
severe headache she had. The older women, however,
have strong praise for their treatement in hospitals
although they do believe their conditions should
have been discovered earlier. Delores, Donna, Ivy
and Ruby in particular complain that doctors in
Britain do not examine women thoroughly enough,
especially when they have gynaecological
complaints.

HEALTH-CARE

There are substantial differences between the groups
over the sorts of health care used. In general,
the Asian women tend to rely on their GPs, whereas
the Afro-Caribbean men prefer to let things heal
naturally without reference to GPs, and the Afro-
Caribbean women tend to use a wealth of home
remedies before they consult a doctor. Home
remedies are not unknown to the Asian women: Reena,
Rajindra and Naseem recall that their parents boiled
up a mixture of herbs to cure a range of illnesses
from stomach complaints to coughs and colds. They
also use preparations available in Britain and the
sub-continent, such as Anadin, Panadol, Benelyn
syrup and Beecham's powders. Otherwise, they
attend their GPs' surgeries, and all but Reena and
Farida had seen a GP within the last six months -
five had seen one during the week before the first
interview.
     The majority (twelve) of the Asian women have
chosen a doctor who can speak Asian languages
because, as Reena says "He can speak our language,
so he can understand our problem". Only four of
the women emphasise that they would prefer a female
doctor, the others wanting just a 'good' doctor.
Eight of the women praise their doctors, but of
these, two (Sufiya and Rajindra) have recently
changed from doctors they were not happy with.
Five women are definitely not satisfied with their
GPs, complaining that they do not spend enough time,
that they treat the people they know better than
others, that they do not try to find out what is
wrong with their patients, and that they are not
sympathetic enough.

130

Black People's Health: A Different Approach

        The   men   of   Afro-Caribbean   descent   are very
critical   of the NHS and GPs in particular.   All of
them   are   extremely sceptical of doctors' abilities
to   effect   cures, and they believe much more in the
power   of   the body's own natural resistance, with a
little   help from some remedies available within the
family.   They   say: "I don't like waitin' when I'm
sick,   I'd   rather   jus'   go   home,   sleep   it off"
(Carlton);   "I   hate doctors . . . If I have a cold
or   a   slight   temperature,   I   would never tell the
doctor,   I   would come here and get some hot ginger or
mint   tea" (Joe);   "I always wait until I have to go
-   really crawling in pain" (Leroy).   Their specific
complaints   are   of   the dinginess of surgeries, the
amount   of   waiting   time,   the   insufficient
consultation   time,   and   the   superiority of the
doctors.   They   prefer to rely on the advice of the
oldest   woman   in   the family in almost all cases of
ill-health,   except   for   accidents   when they use
hospitals.
        The   Afro-Caribbean women talk freely about the
remedies   they   remember   being   used   in their
childhoods   and   some   they   still   use   in Britain
today [40].   Martha,   Delores,   Ruby,   Donna and Ivy
still   use   home remedies before they will consult a
GP,   especially   for   complaints   such as coughs and
colds,   skin rashes, stomach upsets and stiff joints
which   they   feel   doctors are unable to cure.   They
speak   particularly   of the efficacy of herbal teas,
'bay'rum'   (a   cure   for   headaches and fevers), cod
liver malt,   ferrol compounds and a variety of tonics
to   build   the body up.   They tend to have a general
scepticism   about the ability of doctors and drugs to
effect   cures,   and   so   use   them   mainly as a last
resort.   Most of them are not critical of their GPs
per se, but they complain about the lack of time in
the   consultation,   the   automatic   writing out of
prescriptions,   doctors'   failure   to   give adequate
examinations,   and   the   amount of time they have to
wait   before   seeing   their GPs. Consequently, the
women, like the men, tend not to go to see their GPs
very often.
        There   seems   to be a general distrust of drugs
prescribed   by   doctors   in   Britain amongst all the
people   interviewed.   Those from the West Indies, in
particular,   feel that pills cannot do any good, and
they   prefer liquid medicines which they refer to as
'real'   medicine.   Most   of their home remedies are
in   the form of liquids, and these are nearly always
preferred   to   prescribed   tablets.   Even those who

have   found   that tablets are successful in treating
some   conditions are not happy taking them.   Some of
the   Asian women also complain about the prescribing
of   pills.   Several of the older women, taking iron
or   vitamin   tablets,   say that they do not take the
number   of   pills prescribed by their doctor because
they do not think that that number would be good for
them and that too many tablets make them feel 'hot'.
The   concepts   of   'hot'   and 'cold' as they pertain
to   food   and illness are extremely important to the
women   of   Asian   descent as has been found in other
studies [41,42], and   they are also equally relevant
in other cultures.

CONCLUSION

These, then, are some of the preliminary findings of
the   project.   There   are   many   other   sections of
importance   that   could   have   been   included.   The
influence of religion in the majority of the women's
lives,   for example, has been enormous, particularly
in   the way it gives the women strength and peace of
mind   against   the   hardships   and unpleasantness of
everyday   life.   For some of the women, indeed, the
power of prayer to heal illness is seen as much more
potent   than   the power of doctors.   Only Joe of the
men   is actively religious.   The perceived influence
of   food   and   diet   upon   health   is   thought to be
important   by   all   the subjects.   There are some in
both   groups   who   have   managed   to   retain   their
traditional   diets,   but   there   are   others who have
been   affected   by   health education campaigns which
have   attacked   particularly   Asian   diets.   Many of
the   women,   for   example,   find   that   they have to
prepare   western,   usually   'junk'   food   for their
children,   and   many   have incorporated these dishes
into   their own diets.   Some of those who immigrated
to   Britain   criticise   the   value   of   food here,
particularly   the   preponderance   of   processed and
frozen   food,   rather   than   the   fresh   food they
remember from 'back home'.
      The issue of weight is also an interesting one.
The   traditional   ideas from India and Pakistan seem
to   indicate   that   to   be fat is to be healthy, but
this   contrasts   with   the   modern health propaganda
which   declares   the   opposite.   Some   of   the more
overweight Asian women still hold to the traditional
view,   but   the   majority   take   the   middle road,
advocating   a 'sensible' diet and a 'normal' weight.

Black People's Health: A Different Approach

Several of the Afro-Caribbean women are overweight according to their doctors, but they do not think their size is a problem, and it annoys them that their doctors tell them to diet. The younger men and women, however, want to be slim, and dieting and exercise are very important to them.

None of the women of Asian descent has used a hakim or a traditional healer while they have been in Britain. Several of the people of Afro-Caribbean descent prefer private doctors to those working in the NHS. Ivy, Delores, Ruby and Martha have all seen a private doctor, and Donna, Joe, Earl, Danny, Carlton and Paul say they would do so if they were ill because "money talks" (Paul). They feel much more confident that a private doctor would treat them properly and give them thorough examinations because they are paying for the service, and Ivy also claims that their drugs are much more powerful than those on the NHS.

Other important factors include the importance of the effects of depression, loneliness and shock on health, but again and again the preliminary findings of this research show that the focus of much of the previous work in the field of ethnicity and health has little relevance to ordinary black people. The over-concentration on so-called 'exotic' or unusual conditions such as sickle-cell anaemia, rickets and tuberculosis emphasise only negative aspects of black people's health. Only sickle-cell anaemia and thalassaemia actually affect particular ethnic groups because of genetic inheritance, and the numbers who suffer these serious illnesses are actually fewer than white sufferers of cystic fibrosis and haemophilia. Thalassaemia and sickle-cell anaemia deserve attention from medical professionals, but they do not need always to be in the spotlight.

The other conditions generally added to the field of ethnicity and health, such as rickets, tuberculosis, venereal disease and schizophrenia are not complaints specific to particular ethnic groups for genetic reasons, but are probably the result of structural factors affecting minority and usually immigrant populations. Irish and Jewish immigrants suffered similar rates of these illnesses when they first settled in Britain, not because of a racial predeliction for them, but because of the conditions in which they were forced to live [43]. The same is true of black people today. As this research shows, black people, far from being disadvantaged by their race and culture, are able to use traditional

Black People's Health: A Different Approach

and modern patterns and practices as they are
required and to their advantage. Their cultural
inheritances hold many positive elements which can
be employed to improve their health and lives, yet
these have been ignored by researchers.

A new approach to the study of black people's
health has been overdue for some time. There have
been too many studies of 'exotic' diseases, and too
few of lay perceptions of health and illness and the
continued use of traditional patterns and practices.
Similarly, there has been an all too obvious neglect
of the political dimension of black health,
particularly the ways in which racism and racial
discrimination act on black people in all spheres of
life, including health. The new approach to race
and health should seek to combine these two
neglected areas.

REFERENCES

1. Department of Health and Social Security
(1980a) Inequalities in Health: The
Black Report, H.M.S.O., London
2. Townsend, P. and Davidson, N. (1982)
Inequalities in Health, Penguin,
Harmondsworth
3. Donovan, J.L. (1984) Ethnicity and
Health, Social Science and Medicine Vol.
19, pp. 663-670
4. Goel, K.M. (1981) Asians and Rickets,
Lancet, Vol. 2, pp. 405-406
5. British Medical Journal (1978) Rickets,
British Medical Journal, Vol. 1, pp. 804
6. Patterson, S. (1964) Proceedings of the
Royal Society of Medicine, Vol. 57, pp.
325-326
7. Littlewood, R. and Lipsedge, M. (1982)
Aliens and Alienists: Ethnic Minorities
and Psychiatry, Penguin, Harmondsworth
8. Preece, M. et al (1973) Vitamin D
Deficiency, The Lancet, Vol. 1, pp.2
9. British Medical Journal (1978) op. cit.
10. Brent Community Health Council (1981)
Brent People and the Health Service, Brent
CHC, London
11. Goel, K.M. et al (1981) op. cit. pp. 405

12.   Brent CHC (1981) op. cit.
13.   Sheiham,   H.   and   Quick,   A.   (1982) The
        Rickets   Report,   Haringey   CHC   and CRC,
        London
14.   Arneil,   G.   and   Crosbie,   J.   (1963)
        Infantile   Rickets   in   Glasgow,   Lancet,
        Vol. 2,   pp. 423-425
15.   Swan,   C.   and   Cooke,   W.   (1971)
        Nutritional Osteomalacia in immigrants in
        an   urban   community,   Lancet,   Vol. 2,
        pp. 456-459
16.   Department of Health and Social Security
        (1980b)   Rickets   and   Osteomalacia,
        H.M.S.O., London
17.   Community   Relations   Commission   (1976)
        Mental Health Among Minority Groups, CRC,
        London
18.   Rack,   P.   (1979)   Diagnosing   mental
        illness, V. S. Khan (ed) Minority Families
        in Britain, Macmillan, London, pp 165-
        180
19.   Cochrane,   R.   (1979)   Psychological and
        behavioural   disturbance   in West Indians,
        Indians   and   Parkistanis   in   Britain: a
        comparison of rates among children and
        adults,   British Journal of Psychiatry,
        Vol. 14, pp. 201-210
20.   Klein,   R.   (1979) Using the Wrong Label,
        Mind Out, March/April, pp. 16-28
21.   Littlewood,   R.   and   Lipsedge,   M.   (1982)
        op. cit.
22.   Littlewood,   R.   and   Cross,   S.   (1980)
        Ethnic   minorities   and   psychiatric
        services, Sociology of Health and Illness,
        Vol. 2, pp. 2
23.   Torkington, P. (1983) The Racial
        Politics   of   Health,   Department of
        Sociology, Liverpool
24.   Webb,   P.   (1981)   Health   Problems of
        London's   Asians   and   Afro-Caribbeans,
        Health Visitor, Vol. 54, pp. 4
25.   Brent CHC (1981) op. cit.
26.   Fryer,   P.   (1984)   Staying Power,   Pluto
        Press, London
27.   Peach, G.K.C. (1968)   West Indian
        Migration to Britain, Oxford University
        Press, Oxford
28.   Rose, E.J.B. et al (1969) Colour and
        Citizenship,   Institute of Race Relations,
        Oxford University Press, Oxford
29.   Lee,   T.R.   (1977)   Race   and   Residence,
        Clarence Press, Oxford
30.   Smith, D.J. (1977) Racial Disadvantage
        in Britain: The PEP Report, Penguin,
        Harmondsworth

31. Brown, C. (1984) Black and White Britain, Heinemann and Policy Studies Institute, London
32. Doyal, L. (1981) The Political Economy of Health, Pluto Press, London
33. Doyal, L. et al (1983) Cancer in Britain, Pluto Press, London
34. Rose, E. et al (1969) op. cit.
35. Smith, D. (1977) op. cit.
36. Brown, C. (1984) op. cit.
37. Runnymede Trust and Radical Statistics Race Group (1980) Britain's Black Population, Heineman Educational Books, London
38. Sivanandan, A. (1982) A Different Hunger, Pluto Press, London
39. Donovan, J.L. (1983) Black People's Health: A Different Way Forward, Radical Community Medicine, Vol. 6, Winter, pp. 20-29
40. Kitzinger, S. (1980) Women as Mothers: How They See Themselves in Different Cultures, Random House, New York
41. Davies, C. and Aalam, M. (1980) The Hakim and His Role, Rept. to DHSS, London
42. Eagle, R. (1980) Your friendly Neighbourhood Hakim, World Medicine, Vol. 15, pp. 19-22
43. Jones, C. (1977) Immigration and Social Policy in Britain, Tavistock, London

Chapter 6

ETHNIC STATUS AND MENTAL ILLNESS IN URBAN AREAS

John Giggs

INTRODUCTION

In psychiatric epidemiology the identification of
biological, social and environmental correlates of
mental disorders has long constituted a major strand
of both aetiological and health service
research [1]. For social scientists the mental
health implications of a broad range of social
correlates have been matters of sustained interest
since the mid-19th century [2]. Among these diverse
social factors the impact of international migration
and of ethnic status have attracted particular
attention. This is scarcely surprising, because few
nations are now composed entirely of native-born
populations. Indeed, many countries have become
veritable 'melting pots', having attracted
immigrants from all over the world. In the United
States of America (USA) the impact of this
phenomenon was greatest between 1840 and 1920 [3].
In Australia the effects of international migration
have been most marked during the present century,
and 20.2 per cent of the population were classed as
foreign born in 1971 [4]. Even the traditional
'exporting' countries of Europe have also
experienced substantial inflows of migrants in
recent decades. Thus the black immigrant population
of the United Kingdom (UK) has increased from circa
50,000 in 1951 to an estimated 2.2 million in
1980 [5].
    The question of the prevalence of mental
disorders among these burgeoning immigrant
minorities was addressed by pioneer social
scientists as early as the 1840s [6]. Moreover,
large scale <u>scientific</u> investigations of the levels
of mental disorder among native-born and foreign-
born groups have been undertaken since the early
years of the present century [7]. Several recent
literature reviews attest to both the scale and

range of interest in this subject in the USA [8] and the UK [9-11], Europe [12-14] and Australasia [15-19].

The question of the relationship between ethnic status and mental health has been examined in numerous settings in many parts of the world, but the results have frequently been apparently contradictory or inconsistent [20-23]. Furthermore several aspects of the subject have been comparatively briefly explored. This is particularly true of spatial (that is ecological) analyses of ethnic status and mental illness relationships at the intra-urban scale. It is surprising that such studies are relatively rare for, in virtually every country, the immigrant/ethnic minorities are generally disproportionately over-represented in the larger urban settlements. Thus in 1971, 72 per cent of the UK's coloured population (those born in the New Commonwealth and Pakistan) lived in cities with populations of 250,000 or more, compared with only 35 per cent of the total population [24]. Reviews of the relevant inter-urban literature [25,26] also show that most of these ecological studies have been produced by researchers drawn from disciplines for which spatial analysis is not traditionally of great concern. It is extremely regrettable that workers from geography - the one social science in which spatial analysis is the main - should have ignored this field until very recently.

The present chapter therefore focuses upon the main research findings concerning the relationship between ethnic status and mental illness within urban areas. Particular attention is given to the analytical and interpretive problems involved in psychiatric epidemiological research of the ecological level. These problems are viewed in the context of methodological developments which have occurred within the wider fields of urban social geography and medical geography since the early 1960s. The discussion is illustrated with a case study of the incidence and distribution of schizophrenia in the Nottingham Psychiatric Case Register Area. This is an administratively defined unit, comprising the former County Borough of Nottingham and the former Urban Districts of Hucknall, Arnold and Carlton (Figure 6.1). In 1971 the area had a population of 405,661. The Nottingham Psychiatric Case Register (NPCR) was established in 1962 and is one of only eight in the

Figure 6.1:   Residential Mobility, Nottingham 1970–1971

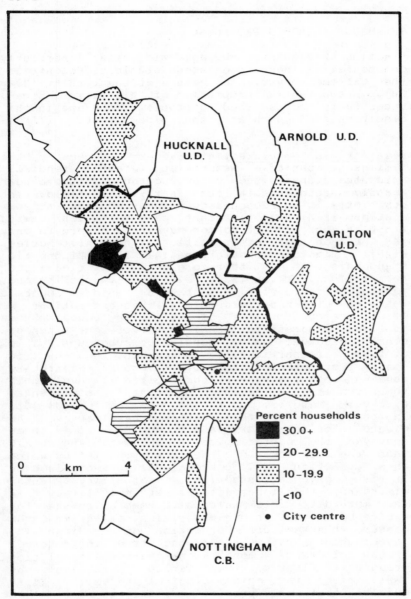

UK (the others are in Aberdeen, Camberwell, Cardiff, Oxford, Salford, Southampton and Worcester).

THE MAJOR RESEARCH PROBLEMS

Existing reviews of the epidemiological literature on mental illness rates among ethnic groups stress the extremely variable nature of the results [27-30]. A substantial proportion of this variation can undoubtedly be ascribed to problems inherent in the disciplines of psychiatry and epidemiology.

Relevant Problems in Psychiatry

Serious comparative scientific research requires accurate standardised data but such data are not readily obtained in this particular field. In psychiatry it is recognised that marked temporal and spatial (regional, international) variations exist in both the classification of mental disorders and the recognition of specific illness categories within diagnosed populations [31,32]. Diagnostic standardisation is therefore still a crucial issue for clinical workers [33] and seriously inhibits the possibilities of comparative epidemiological research between different localities and nations.

A second source of variation concerns the problems inherent in identifying different kinds of mental disorder among population subgroups. This problem is particularly acute in the specific context of ethnic groups. Numerous researchers have demonstrated the cultural pitfalls involved in the recognition of several important forms of mental disorder among immigrant ethnic minorities [34-37]. In the UK many ethnic patients have received the diagnosis of schizophrenia although " . . . it often conveyed the doctor's lack of understanding rather than the presence of the 'key symptoms' by which this reaction is conventionally recognised by British psychiatrists" [38]. For many mental disorders, therefore, it is extremely likely that the morbidity rates which have been calculated for native-born and ethnic minorities reflect in large measure the culture perceptions of the diagnosing psychiatrists rather than the 'true' incidence of these disorders among these various population groups. Clearly this issue has important implications for epidemiological research. It is evident that the problem is likely to be resolved only where psychiatrists have received appropriate training and considerable experience in diagnosing and treating mental disorders in ethnic populations.

Both the levels and kinds of mental disorders found in the general population are also determined to a significant extent by nosocomial (that is health service related) factors. In most countries case-finding and recording methods vary markedly between localities, resulting in widely contrasting levels of psychiatric morbidity in the populations studied. Since the early 1950s the range of mental health services in most western countries has been extended to include not only the large traditional in-patient and community based psychiatric services [39,40]. Unfortunately, marked regional variations have developed in the extent to which these new services have been adopted, especially within the UK [41]. Consequently the contacts with psychiatric services in one locality in the UK may be derived almost exclusively from hospital in-patient records, whereas those from another locality (for example, the NPCR Area) have been acquired over a very broad range of psychiatric services. These dramatic regional variations in the range of psychiatric services affect not only the levels of mental disorder determined for the whole population, but also for important groups, such as ethnic minorities and the elderly, since these appear to be picked up with contrasting levels of efficiency by different components of the psychiatric health care service system [42-46].

The range, quality and reliability of data relating to patients's characteristics also tend to vary markedly between psychiatric registers. With respect to ethnic minorities these phenomena are of particular importance. In recent years several authors have commented on the problem of the unavailability of information on country of birth [47,48]. In an analysis of mental hospital admissions for the whole of England and Wales during 1971 Cochrane [49] reported that information on country of birth was missing for 30 per cent of all patients. It would appear to be the case that the gaps result largely from the failure of (register) staff to record the birth place of British and Irish-born persons. Similar inaccuracies frequently appear for persons born in particular countries. Thus patients often give their birth place as 'Ireland' without specifying whether they mean the Republic or Northern Ireland.

The limitations of psychiatric register information for patients extend beyond the accuracy of birth place information. In the case of the NPCR only 60 per cent of all persons contacting services for the first time during 1969-73 had details concerning occupation entered on their records. In the particular case of the first admission schizophrenics identified during the same period 15 per cent were subsequently found to have given home addresses which were either non-existent or incorrect. Whatever the causes, these incomplete (and often erroneous) data files require cautious handling if accurate statistics are to be produced.

Relevant Epidemiological Problems

The difficulties outlined briefly above are compounded by those specific to psychiatric epidemiology. These derive from the characteristics of the numerator (the mentally ill population), the denominator (the host, or base, population) and the particular methodology used to calculate rates of mental disorder. The lack of comparability in the choice of elements used in psychiatric epidemiological studies of mental disorders among ethnic minorities and host populations makes accurate comparision a difficult task.

The numerator data bases used by different authors tend to vary markedly in character and comprehensiveness. They range from a few rare community surveys, to analyses of general practitioner records or of entire psychiatric register services (such as hospital in patients, out patients, day patients, clinic attendances and domiciliary visits). The majority of investigations, however, are based exclusively upon psychiatric hospital admissions [50]. Even here, important methodological differences can be identified. Some workers have calculated illness rates by using only first admission cases for a specified period whilst others have used unduplicated admissions (that is first admissions and unduplicated readmissions during a year), or total admissions. Some authors have used all three data bases to calculate hospital admission rates for minority groups and native-born persons [51].

It is generally recognised that ethnic minorities are extremely variegated and differ from the majority in terms of birthplace, race, language, religion and other important cultural traits [52,53]. Unfortunately both psychiatric registers and national population censuses provide information for only a limited range of these attributes. Consequently it is not possible to calculate accurate morbidity rates for many important population groups. The UK population censuses have been especially unsatisfactory in this respect [54,55]. Only three tables relating to ethnic minority groups were published in the 1971 census. The first simply identified two broad groups of residents with neither parent born in the UK (that is those with 'both parents born in the New Commonwealth' and 'others'!). These were further subdivided into eight age bands and by sex and marital status. Only two marital status categories were identified and they therefore contained important subgroups which are significantly over represented among the populations which use psychiatric services. Thus the 'married' category apparently also includes persons who are separated. Similarly the second marital status category - SWD (single, widowed and divorced) also groups together three distinct yet potentially important precipitants of mental disorder [56]. These blunt census instruments therefore conceal important and growing segments of the population in Western countries [57].

The second census table relating to ethnic groups identified ethnicity simply in terms of birth places (country of birth). For non-UK born residents sex is reported for only eleven broad birth place categories in the Small Area Census Tabulations (see Table 6.5). The geographical areas identified are mostly extremely large and several obviously aggregate populations from many different countries (such as the Old Commonwealth and Europe). Moreover, since no information on age is provided for these groups, it is not possible to calculate accurate age-adjusted morbidity rates for mental disorders. This is a very important limitation because there are marked variations in the age profiles of the major ethnic groups living in the UK [58,59]. For important mental disorders like schizophrenia (found mainly in 15-30 year olds) and the senile psychoses (found mainly in the over 65s) the distorting effects of using crude total population figures are bound to be substantial.

The data presented in the third table relating to ethnicity in the 1971 census was even more highly

aggregated.   It identified the birthplaces of those
entering   the   UK after 1960.   These were classified
by   sex   for   only   five   'geographical' areas - the
Irish   Republic,   the   Old Commonwealth,   the New
Commonwealth,   Other   Europe and a residual category
(Other   Foreign and Not Stated).   Unfortunately this
information   is   of   little   use   in   psychiatric
epidemiological   research.   The geographical groups
are too highly aggregated and the time span involved
(1960-71)   is   really too great to test the temporal
relationships   between timing of migration and onset
of   mental   disorder which have been demonstrated so
effectively   in   Australian   and   North   American
studies [60,61].

Relevant Problems in Ecological Analysis

In   the   introductory   section   it   was   noted that
although   immigrant/ethnic   minorities   are
disproportionately   concentrated   within   urban
settlements   in   most   countries,   comparatively few
studies   exist   which measure the spatial patterning
of   these   groups,   their   mental   illness rates and
their   relationships   with   environmental   factors.
The shortcomings of the use of the terms 'immigrant'
and   'ethnic'   as   interchangeable were also noted in
Chapter   1.   These   issues have been intermittently
examined by several workers since the publication of
Faris   and   Dunham's classic analysis of the spatial
distribution   of mental   disorders   in Chicago [62].
However, the ecological approach which they espoused
has   continued   to   occupy an essentially peripheral
position   in   psychiatric   epidemiological research.
Furthermore,   the   majority of workers in this field
have   apparently remained unaware of the substantial
and   relevant   theoretical   and   methodological
contributions   to   the broader field of urban social
ecology   which   have   been made by social scientists
since the early 1960s.
     When   the   existing   psychiatric   ecological
studies   are   examined   within   the context of these
developments   their   limitations and diverse results
are   better   understood.   One   important   source of
variation   arises   from   the   fact   that urban
settlements within Western countries differ markedly
from   each other in terms of such critical variables
as   age   of   the   city,   population   size,   economic
structure   and   social composition [63-67].   This
marked   variability   in   general characteristics is
matched   by   equally wide differences between cities
in   terms of the growth rates, size and diversity of

their resident ethnic groups [68,69]. These marked variations in contextual attributes have substantial implications for ethnic minorities, in terms of their settlement histories, patterns and mental health.

Variations in the results of psychiatric epidemiological studies of ethnic groups can also be partly ascribed to the fact that no uniform areal definition of urban settlements has been adopted. Several kinds of boundaries have been used, with consequent implications for the results which have emerged. Thus some authors have examined only the urban administrative area level [70], whereas others have examined the urban-suburban level [71]. Still others have analysed urban-rural differentials [72].

The diversity of the choice of size of study area has been exceeded by the adoption of an even more variegated range of areal sub-units within study areas. These have ranged in size from street blocks at the lower end of the spectrum [73] to entire Metropolitan Boroughs at the upper end [74]. The contrasting sizes of the basic areal 'building blocks' used in intra-urban studies produce statistically significant variations in the results of epidemiological analyses [75]. They also influence the levels of spatial segregation obtained for ethnic groups. In a recent review of the subject Boal has stated that "the scale of data sub-sets employed in a segregation study can fundamentally influence the values for segregation indices obtained. The smaller the size of the data sub-sets the longer the segregation index values" [76]. This factor is clearly of great importance since contrasting levels of social and spatial propinquity have frequently been cited as reasons for spatial variations in the incidence of mental disorders among ethnic minorities living in cities [77].

A further serious limitation of existing ecological psychiatric investigations stems from the fact that they are almost all uniformly cross-sectional in character. Consideration is rarely given to the effects of temporal facts. Virtually every study is based upon an analysis of rates of mental disorder calculated for relevant populations living in a specified set of areas at one particular census date, and in some instances this strategy has probably seriously distorted the results. Faris and Dunham [78], for example, aggregated mental hospital admissions in Chicago for the two periods 1922-31, 1922-34 and calculated rates for the total

population, foreign-born persons, and for negroes
and other races, using the 1930 population census as
the source for the denominator populations.
Unfortunately, during the period 1920-30, all these
population groups changed considerably in size
(Table 6.1).

Table 6.1: Chicago's Population, by Race and
Nativity

	1920	1930	Per cent change
	(000s)		
Total population	2,702	3,376	+24.9
Native white			
native parentage	643	943	+46.7
foreign/mixed	1,141	1,332	+16.7
parentage	1,141	1,332	+16.7
Foreign-born white	805	842	+4.6
Negro and other races	113	259	+129.2

Source: US Bureau of the Census (1941).
Statistical Abstract of the United States: 1940,
Washington DC.

Furthermore, these substantial aggregate
changes mask considerable intra-urban variations in
the rates and direction of population turnover.
Thus most inner city neighbourhoods have lost
population while suburban areas have grown. Big
changes can occur within city neighbourhoods over
quite short periods of time and in the USA
approximately 20 per cent of households move home
every year, compared with 7-12 per cent in the
UK [79]. In the 1971 census 12.3 per cent of all
the households living in the NPCR Area were reported
to have changed residence within the previous year.
Figure 6.1 shows that there were also considerable
spatial variations in the levels of household
mobility within the study area. This issue is of
particular importance when relatively small but fast
growing and mobile population groups such as ethnic
minorities are being examined. Recent reviews of
the literature have shown that the spatial outcomes
of ethnic minority settlement within cities are
often extremely fluid and variable [80-82].

ETHNICITY AND SCHIZOPHRENIA IN NOTTINGHAM

Although the subject of mental illness among ethnic minorities has long attracted both popular and academic interest, many important aspects remain unclear and unresolved. The discussion presented above showed that several problems relevant to the subject persist within the fields of clinical psychiatry, psychiatric epidemiology and ecological psychiatry. These have considerable implications both for data analysis and interpretation of the results. The following case study of ethnicity and schizophrenia in Nottingham exemplified these issues.

The Study Area and its Population
The area chosen for examination is served by the NPCR. It is an administratively defined unit, comprising the city of Nottingham and three contiguous Urban Districts (Figure 6.1). In 1971 the city was ranked ninth in population size among urban settlements in England and Wales. The Register area contained the bulk of the population of the spatially more extensive Nottingham metropolitan area defined by Hall et al [83]. In 1971 the employment structure was typically metropolitan for only 41.9 per cent of all employed persons worked in manufacturing industry (chiefly textiles and engineering). By contrast, the census occupation tables showed that only 24.2 per cent of the workforce was actually employed in manufacturing.

The demographic and socio-economic structure of the NPCR area differed from the national picture in several important respects (Table 6.2). The age structure of the population was slightly younger than that for the whole of England and Wales. The socio-economic profile of the working male population was heavily weighted in the skilled and semi-skilled manual categories. The structure of the area's tenure system reflected this character, for the proportion of owner occupied property was much lower than the national average.

The population size of the NPCR area changed relatively little between 1951 and 1971. Over the two decades it increased by only 5.4 per cent, compared with 11.4 per cent for England and Wales. Between 1961 and 1971 the County Borough began to lose population to the contiguous suburban areas (Table 6.3) and to the rural districts outside the study area [84].

Table 6.2:   NPCR Area Selected Demographic and
Housing Traits: 1971

A.   Population Age Structure (per cent)

	Nottingham	England and Wales
0-14	24.9	23.7
15-24	15.4	14.5
25-34	11.4	12.4
35-44	11.6	11.7
45-54	12.5	12.4
55-64	11.8	11.9
65+	12.2	13.4

B.   Socio-economic Groups, Males (per cent)

		Nottingham	England and Wales
1.	Professional etc	12	17
2.	Other non-manual	16	18
3.	Skilled manual	44	39
4.	Semi-skilled manual	17	15
5.	Unskilled manual	11	11

C. Housing Tenure Categories (per cent)

		Nottingham	England and Wales
1.	Owner occupied	35.2	51.1
2.	L.A. rented	39.5	28.1
3.	Rented unfurnished	21.4	16.7
4.	Rented furnished	3.6	3.7
5.	Other	0.3	0.4

Source: 1971 Census Population and Economic
Activity Tables

Table 6.3: NPCR Area Population Structure and
Change, 1961-71

	1961	1971	Per cent change
Nottingham P.R.A.	400,812	405,661	1.2
City	311,899	300,630	-3.6
Suburbs	88,913	105,031	18.1
Arnold U.D.	26,829	33,422	24.6
Carlton U.D.	38,815	45,235	16.5
Hucknall U.D.	23,269	26,374	13.3

Source: 1971 Census. Nottinghamshire County
Report.

The losses experienced by the City were partially
offset by a substantial increase in the foreign-born
population. Unfortunately, detailed figures of the
numbers and birthplaces of these immigrants were
only published for Nottingham C.B. The three urban
districts which make up the fringe of the NPCR area
each had populations of less than 50,000 and were
therefore omitted from the published statistics.
However, a reasonably accurate assessment of
changing numbers and composition can be obtained
from the existing census information because, even
as late as 1971, the bulk of the foreign-born
population (87.0 per cent) lived within Nottingham
C.B. The unpublished Small Area Statistics census
tabulations provided data on birthplace for the
entire study area for 1971.
    Table 6.4 summarises the main changes which
occurred within the foreign-born resident population
of Nottingham C.B. between 1951 and 1971. It shows
that the substantial increase in the total number of
foreign-born persons over the two decades could be
attributed chiefly to those coming from three main
sources within the New Commonwealth and Pakistan
(NCWP) block - the West Indies (88 per cent of these
were Jamaicans), India and Pakistan. The Irish-born
population almost doubled between 1951 and 1961, but
declined slightly thereafter. By contrast, the
numbers of European-born persons remained fairly
constant over the whole period. However, there
were quite pronounced changes in the composition of
the European-born population. For example, the
numbers from Eastern European countries declined
substantially, whereas those from Common Market
countries increased.

149

Table 6.4:   Growth of the Foreign Born Population
in Nottingham C.B. 1951-1971

	1951	1961	1971
Total foreign-born	11,193	16,192	21,675
West Indies	98	3,305	5,421
India	497	996	2,250
Pakistan	85	362	1,790
Eire[a]	2,476	4,261	3,990
Europe	5,198	5,787	5,770
Poland	2,306	2,095	1,725
U.S.S.R.	1,303	1,227	1,205
Italy	103	880	1,090

[a] includes Irish, not stated (i.e. whether
from Irish Republic or Northern Ireland)

Sources: Population Census Nottinghamshire
County Reports, 1951 1961, 1971.

The major demographic attributes of the foreign-born
population of the entire study area in 1971 are
summarised in Table 6.5.   The NCWP source is
clearly dominant in the local context.   Jones [85]
notes that Nottingham C.B. ranked ninth among the
urban settlements of England and Wales in numbers of
immigrants from this source.   Five groups –
Europeans, Irish, West Indians, Indians and
Pakistanis – accounted for 79.7 per cent of the
total foreign-born population.

The Incidence of Schizophrenia in Nottingham
The first part of the psychiatric epidemiological
investigation comprised a retrospective examination
of the case notes of all contacts with all
psychiatric services in the NPCR area during the
five year period 1969-73.   Attention was restricted
to first contact cases with a primary diagnosis of
schizophrenia or paranoia (International
Classification of Diseases [ICD], codes 295 and
297) and aged between 15 and 59 years.   The cases
were initially differentiated by sex and birthplace.
A further distinction was made between cases living
at private addresses and those from non-private
addresses (hostels and hotels) and of no fixed abode
(Table 6.6).

Ethnic Status and Mental Illness in Urban Areas

Table 6.5: Birthplace of Present Residents in the NPCR Area: 1971

	Males	Females	% Female	Total	% Total
Irish Republic	2,256	2,114	48.4	4,370	1.1
Old Commonwealth	269	247	47.9	516	0.1
New Commonwealth	5,974	4,918	45.7	10,892	2.8
Africa	379	253	40.0	632	0.2
America (W. Indies)	2,756	2,716	49.6	5,481	1.4
Ceylon	23	17	42.5	40	---
India	1,251	1,044	45.5	2,295	0.6
Pakistan	1,209	574	32.2	1,783	0.5
Far East	185	150	44.7	335	0.1
Remainder	165	160	49.2	325	0.1
Other European	2,735	3,186	53.8	5,921	1.5
Other Foreign Not Stated	1,933	1,276	39.8	3,209	0.8
Total Foreign Born	13,167	11,741	47.1	24,908	6.5
UK Born	174,509	185,921	51.6	360,430	93.5
Total	187,676	197,662	51.3	385,338	100.0

Source: Population Census, 1971. Small Area Statistics

Table 6.6: First Contacts with Psychiatric Services in the NPCR Area by Sex, Birthplace and Residential Status: 1969-73

	Total Cases		Residents		Non-residents	
	M	F	M	F	M	F
UK-born	153	166	119	96	34	20
Foreign-born	65	49	54	46	11	3
Irish	21	14	16	12	5	2
European	17	13	13	13	4	0
Old Commonwealth	1	1	0	1	1	0
Other Foreign	0	2	0	1	0	1
New Commonwealth	26	19	25	19	1	0
West Indian	15	15	15	15	0	0
Indian	8	4	8	4	0	0
Pakistani	2	0	2	0	0	0
Total cases	218	165	173	142	45	23

Source: Nottingham Psychiatric Case Register

The results of the analysis were dramatic. Although foreign-born persons accounted for only 6.5 per cent of the total population in 1971 (Table 6.5), they constituted 29.8 per cent of all the cases (Table 6.6). This compares very closely with the figure of 29.2 per cent identified for the period 1963-69 in an earlier study of the incidence of first contacts in Nottingham C.B. [86]. Table 6.6 also reveals that substantial proportions of the cases were not living at private addresses at the time of first contact (total cases 17.8 per cent, UK-born cases 20.1 per cent, all foreign-born cases 12.3 per cent). This substantial element in the client population consisted chiefly of 'drifters', most of whom were not local residents. They clearly inflate the numbers of total first contacts quite considerably. Unfortunately it is difficult to assess their significance in other localities because most workers have not identified this particular group in the analysis of admission rates. Intuitively one would expect their numbers to be higher in large cities than in smaller urban settlements.

The incidence rates of schizophrenia (ICD 295 and 297 combined) for the major ethnic groups are presented in Table 6.7. The rates were calculated for all cases and for residents. A comparison of the relevant columns (1 and 3) confirms that the rates among the Irish-born and European-born populations fall markedly when residential status is considered. The annual rates for the total male and female populations fall within the range of 15-20 per 100,000 population at risk recognised by Wing [87]. Among the resident foreign-born groups (column 3) the rates for persons born in the Old Commonwealth, Other Foreign Countries and Pakistan are generally low and clearly influenced by the small numbers involved. Among the Irish, Europeans, West Indians and Indians the rates are all considerably higher than those for British-born persons.

There are many contributory factors which account for the enormous disparities between the rates for the British-born population and those for most of the foreign-born groups. The specific effects of social class and age structure cannot be measured since appropriate census data are not available. Similarly the impact of marital status and family setting upon both the development of schizophrenia and probability of contact with psychiatric services cannot be assessed. Several

Table 6.7: Average Annual Incidence of Schizophrenia in
the NPCR Area by Birthplace, 1969-73

(Rate per 100,000 persons)

MALES

	All Cases[a]		Residents only	
	Total[b]	Schizophrenics[c]	Total[b]	Schizophrenics[c]
UK-born	17.5	10.0	13.6	8.9
Foreign-born	98.7	66.8	82.0	56.2
Irish	186.2	115.2	141.8	106.4
European	124.3	65.8	95.1	51.2
Old Commonwealth	74.3	74.3	0	0
Other Foreign	0	0	0	0
New Commonwealth	87.0	70.3	83.7	60.3
West Indian	108.5	79.6	108.5	79.6
Indian	127.9	111.9	127.9	111.9
Pakistani	33.1	33.1	33.1	33.1
Total population	23.2	14.0	18.4	10.6

FEMALES

	All Cases[a]		Residents only	
	Total[b]	Schizophrenics[c]	Total[b]	Schizophrenics[c]
UK-born	12.5	8.0	10.3	7.5
Foreign-born	83.5	49.4	78.4	49.9
Irish	132.5	94.6	113.5	94.6
European	81.6	37.7	81.6	37.7
Old Commonwealth	81.0	81.0	81.0	81.0
Other Foreign	31.0	15.7	15.7	15.7
New Commonwealth	77.3	44.7	77.3	44.7
West Indian	110.4	51.5	110.4	51.5
Indian	76.6	76.6	76.6	76.6
Pakistani	0	0	0	0
Total population	16.7	10.4	14.4	10.0

[a] Includes both cases living in private addresses and those living in
     hostels, hotels or of no fixed abode.
[b] Includes Schizophrenics (ICD 295) and Paranoid Cases (ICD 297).
[c] Schizophrenics only (ICD 295), excluding paranoid schizophrenics
     (ICD 295.3)

workers have suggested that the high rates of schizophrenia found among foreign-born persons might be attributable to certain transcultural factors and behaviour patterns which might tend to both increase the likelihood of contact with psychiatric services and produce a diagnosis of schizophrenia [88,89]. These behaviour patterns might increase the likelihood of such diagnosis as paranoia and paranoid schizophrenia (ICD 297 and ICD 295.3). This possibility was examined in the Nottingham data by calculating incidence rates of non-paranoid schizophrenia for all the population groups. The results are summarised in Table 6.7 (columns 2 and 4). The data reveal that, even when allowance is made for these diagnostic factors, the rates for most of the foreign-born groups remain considerably higher than those for the British-born population. However, the subject of diagnostic consistency still deserves to be examined in further detail, particularly within the context of the residential histories and family settings of the different ethnic groups. The NCWP population is characterised by a 'young' age profile and by a matching profile among the schizophrenic cohort (66.6. per cent of the cases were aged 15-34). Furthermore, the bulk of the NCWP population could be classed as recent settlers since 58.3 per cent had arrived in the Register Area between 1960 and 1971. By contrast, the Irish and European groups have 'older' age profiles, both among their total populations and the schizophrenics (54.2 per cent of Irish-born cases and only 16.7 per cent of European-born cases were aged 15-34). Most of the Irish and European populations have also lived in Nottingham for a considerable period of time and only 18.0 per cent of the Irish and 19.4 per cent of the European populations had settled in Nottingham after 1960.

Schizophrenia and the Ecological Structure of Nottingham

Considerable problems still exist, therefore, in both clinical psychiatry and psychiatric epidemiology concerning the issues of diagnostic standardisation, case identification and the calculation of accurate rates of mental disorder among native-born and immigrant or ethnic groups. Despite these problems the fact that the incidence rates for most mental disorders apparently vary considerably between population groups is of particular interest to researchers involved in ecological psychiatry, for these groups are generally unevenly distributed within large urban settlements [90-93].

Recent reviews of the ecological literature demonstrate that several studies have addressed the particular issues of both the spatial variations in the distribution of mental disorders among ethnic groups within cities and their social/environmental correlates [94,95]. The explication of the methodological limitations of existing psychiatric ecological research presented in the first section of this paper showed that there is considerable scope for further research in this particular field. The data obtained for Nottingham provide an opportunity to exemplify some of the relevant methodological developments which have occurred in urban social ecology and medical geography since the early 1960s.

The most important technical decision in ecological research is the choice of an appropriate set of areal units to form the spatial framework for subsequent data analysis. Ideally these should bound the limits of the 'true' social-environmental areas within the city. Unfortunately this requirement is rarely satisfied since researchers have been obliged to use the existing territorial divisions delineated by census officers for the collection and analysis of census data. Faris and Dunham [96], for example used 120 census-based 'sub-community areas' in their pioneer analysis of mental disorders in Chicago. They selected seven census variables and used these to aggregate the 120 areas into eleven distinct types of 'natural area' within the city.

A second important requirement in the selection of the spatial framework is that the number of areas used should be related to the number of cases (for example hospital admissions) being studied. In several studies the particular scale adopted has produced results which are not particularly enlightening. In Levy and Rowitz' [97] study of Chicago 75 Community Areas were used to calculate age-adjusted rates for only 131 first admission senile and arteriosclerotic cases and 197 manic depressives. At the other end of the scale Hare based his analysis of the ecological patterning of schizophrenia in Bristol on only three areas, each comprising five electoral wards [98]. He also excluded four wards from his analysis on the grounds that they were "notably heterogeneous as regards social characteristics" [99].

In the present study of the NPCR area fifteen distinct social-environmental areas were employed. These were obtained from a Principal Components Analysis and a non-hierarchical cluster analysis of 62 census variables for the 796 enumeration districts located within the NPCR area in 1971. A full account of this analysis is given elsewhere [100]. These multivariate statistical methods produced a comprehensive and objective picture of the 'ecological' areas which existed in the study area in 1971. Their key attributes are summarised via brief descriptive labels in Table 6.8 and their spatial distribution is shown in Figures 6.2A-6.2D.

The ethnic minorities resident in the NPCR area are very unevenly distributed geographically. Table 6.8 and Figures 6.3A-6.3B give general impressions of their aggregated distributions in 1971. For all foreign born residents the pattern is dominated by a sector extending north from the city centre (Figure 6.3B). This is the classic immigrant/transient area (Table 6.8, areas 1 and 2). Beyond this central sector the rates of foreign-born representation in the total population decline more or less zonally with increasing distance from the city centre. The proportions of recent migrants among the foreign-born populations present a broadly similar pattern (Table 6.8, column 4). Figure 6.3A shows the distribution of the population with both parents foreign born. Because the numbers involved are larger than those in the more limited foreign-born category, secondary localised concentrations appear in the cores of the three suburban Urban Districts and in north Nottingham.

The general patterns shown in Figures 6.3A-6.3B and Table 6.8 conceal substantial variations in the spatial distributions of the major ethnic groups living in Nottingham. Given the considerable differences in both the numbers and phasing of immigration among the major ethnic groups, considerable variations existed in their levels of spatial segregation by 1971. These spatial variations are summarised in Table 6.9. Here the rates for each ethnic group in each of the fifteen ecological areas are presented as ratios of their per cent representation in the whole study area (Table 6.5, column 5). For the four ethnic groups identified the spatial pattern is similar to that for the entire foreign-born population (classically zonal), with rates declining progressively outwards from the city centre. For the longer settled Irish

Table 6.8:   Selected Demographic Attributes of the Ecological Areas in the NPCR Area 1971

		Total Population	Total Foreign-born	Foreign-born of total	Recent[a] Migrants
Inner city, low status					
1.	Immigrant/ transient core	1.9	9.4	33.6	48.8
2.	Immigrant/ transient frame	3.8	11.3	20.3	38.6
3.	Early family	7.1	16.1	15.5	44.7
4.	Ageing family	13.3	19.8	10.1	38.1
Inner city, high status					
5.	Transient	1.2	2.2	12.2	33.9
Middle city, middle status					
6.	Aged family housing	12.4	8.2	4.4	19.9
7.	Established/ ageing family	13.8	9.9	4.8	22.7
Outer city, high status					
8.	New/established family	7.0	3.6	3.4	21.9
9.	Ageing family	5.4	4.0	5.0	15.3
10.	University	0.8	0.4	3.9	83.2
Outer city, council estates					
11.	Low status, new family	2.3	2.6	7.4	29.3
12.	Low status, mature family	6.0	3.0	3.4	24.5
13.	Low status, ageing family	8.0	3.0	2.5	20.3
14.	Middle status, mature family	10.2	4.3	2.8	17.2
15.	Middle status, mixed family	5.8	2.3	2.3	14.6
	Total	100.0	100.0	6.5	33.8

[a] Per cent of foreign-born population entering the UK during 1960-71

Figure 6.2: Distribution of the Demographic Attributes of the Ecological Areas in the NPCR Area

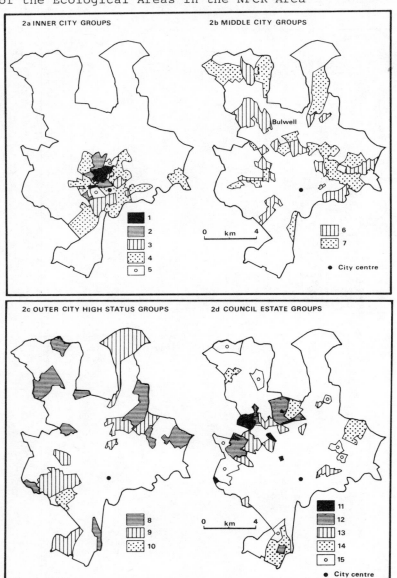

Ethnic Status and Mental Illness in Urban Areas

Figure 6.3: Distribution of Major Ethnic Groups
within the NPCR Area

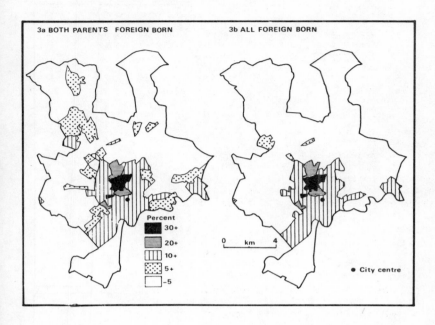

159

Table 6.9: Distribution of the Major Ethnic Groups Within the NPCR Area 1971
            (Standardised Rates [a])

Clusters	Total	Eire	Europe	West Indies	India/ Pakistan
Inner city, low status					
1. Immigrant/ transient core	517	229	265	765	991
2. Immigrant/ transient frame	312	240	261	326	420
3. Early family	238	222	118	266	379
4. Ageing family	155	141	124	201	152
Inner city, high status					
5. Transient	188	152	282	44	157
Middle city, middle status					
6. Aged family/housing	68	68	104	39	27
7. Established/ageing family	74	71	118	35	42
Outer city, high status					
8. New/established family	52	62	72	12	25
9. Ageing family	77	87	123	12	36
10. University	60	76	51	21	14
Outer city, council estates					
11. Low status, new family	114	77	52	306	17
12. Low status, mature family	52	71	32	68	8
13. Low status, ageing family	38	66	59	23	9
14. Middle status, mature family	43	51	52	15	7
15. Middle status, mixed family	35	64	39	20	12

[a] Nottingham P.C.R. area total = 100

and European groups the range of variation in rates
is relatively slight. Among the recently settled
West Indians, Indians and Pakistanis, however, the
gradients are extremely steep. These ethnic groups
are massively concentrated in the low status inner
city areas. The reasons for the emergence of this
particular pattern of residential segregation among
NCP immigrants in Nottingham have been fully
documented elsewhere [101-103].

The uneven spatial concentration of ethnic
groups within the study area has potentially
important repercussions for the ecological analysis
of the distribution patterns of schizophrenics,
since it has already been established that the
incidence of the disorder is apparently much greater
among immigrant groups than the native-born
population. In many ecological investigations of
the incidence of the disorder within urban areas the
schizophrenic population has been treated as an
undifferentiated (aggregated) group. In these
studies the spatial patterning of incidence rates
has typically been zonal, with the highest rates
occurring in the central areas and the lowest in the
suburbs. The distribution of standardised rates
within the NPCR area also accords broadly with this
stereotype (Figure 6.4A). The statistical
probability that these rates could have occurred by
change can be measured, using the Poisson
formula [104]. Figure 6.4B also shows the areas in
which the rates of schizophrenia were higher (or
lower) than expected at the 0.5 level.

When the total schizophrenic population of the
study area is differentiated according to birthplace
(Table 6.10) it becomes evident that the foreign-
born cases are strongly over-represented in the four
low status inner-city areas and in one of the
suburban council estate groups (group 13 - low
status, ageing family).

The distribution of standardised rates of
schizophrenia for the total foreign-born population
(Table 6.11, column 3 and Figure 6.5) presents a
rather complex picture. Although the low status
inner city areas have quite high rates the highest
concentrations are found in the scattered low
status, ageing family, group of council estates
(Group 13). Probability analysis (Figure 6.5)
shows that only the Group 13 council estates have
rates which are greater than might be expected by
chance. The data presented in Table 6.9, however,
showed that the foreign-born persons constituted
only a very small proportion of the total population

Figure 6.4:   Distribution of Total Schizophrenic Cases

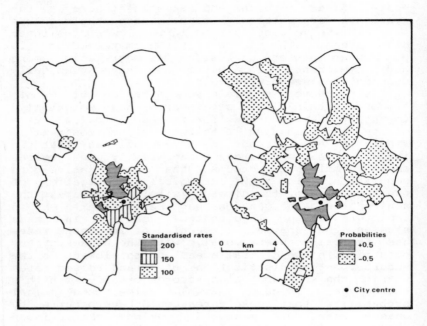

Ethnic Status and Mental Illness in Urban Areas

Table 6.10: Distribution of Schizophrenics [a], by Birthplace, in the NPCR
Area 1969-73

	Total	Foreign-born	Foreign-born as % of total
Inner city, low status			
1. Immigrant/transient core	21	13	61.9
2. Immigrant/transient frame	29	16	55.2
3. Early family	31	19	61.3
4. Ageing family	47	25	53.2
Inner city, high status			
5. Transient	5	1	20.0
Middle city, high status			
6. Aged family/housing	39	4	10.3
7. Established/ageing family	33	9	27.3
Outer city, high status			
8. New/established family	15	0	0
9. Ageing family	14	2	14.2
10. University	3	0	0
Outer city, council estates			
11. Low status, new family	10	0	0
12. Low status, mature family	15	2	13.3
13. Low status, ageing family	13	6	46.2
14. Middle status, mature family	22	2	9.1
15. Middle status, mixed family	18	1	5.6
Total	315	100	30.8

[a] Persons resident in private dwellings and having a diagnosis of
Schizophrenia (ICD 295) or paranoia (ICD 297)

Table 6.11: Distribution of Rates of Schizophrenia, by Birthplace, in the NPCR Area (Standardised Rates [a])

	Total	Native-born	Foreign-born	Eire	Europe	West Indies	India/Pakistan
Inner city, low status							
1. Immigrant/transient core	314	34	138	141	156	117	179
2. Immigrant/transient frame	243	186	155	174	40	220	106
3. Early family	150	97	116	153	60	106	61
4. Ageing family	123	88	126	114	189	89	124
Inner city, high status							
5. Transient	98	122	47	0	0	636	
6. Aged family/housing	105	133	50	77	61	0	0
7. Established/ageing family	75	77	87	33	143	71	0
Outer city, high status							
8. New/established family	64	88	0	0	0	0	0
9. Ageing family	82	98	61	70	59	0	0
10. University	75	104	0	0	0	0	0
Outer city, council estates							
11. Low status, new family	127	182	0	0	0	0	0
12. Low status, mature family	83	99	93	0	202	83	0
13. Low status, ageing family	57	42	292	72	253	205	880
14. Middle status, mature family	66	83	50	50	64	0	0
15. Middle status, mixed family	75	96	47	0	111	0	0

[a] Nottingham PCR area total = 100

Figure 6.5:   Distribution of Foreign Born Cases

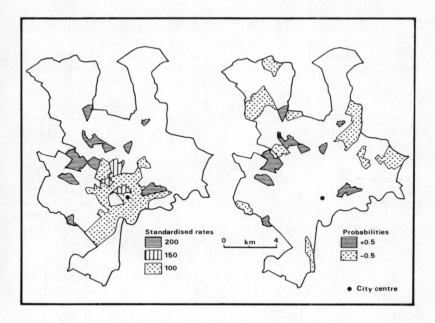

in these estates. When the total foreign-born schizophrenic population is disaggregated into its constituent ethnic groups (Table 6.11, columns 4-7) it can be seen that the high rate has been created by cases born in Europe, the West Indies and India/Pakistan. This phenomenon has been identified in a number of urban ecological analyses of the incidence of schizophrenia. In Chicago both Faris and Dunham [105] and Levy and Rowitz [106] found that the rates of shizophrenia were substantially higher among blacks living in areas where they formed a minority of the total population rather than in areas where they constituted the majority.

When all native-born schizophrenics are examined as a subset of the total schizophrenic population their spatial distribution also presents distinctive characteristics. Figure 6.6 and Table 6.11 (column 2) reveal that rates in excess of the average are scattered throughout the study area. Probability analysis and mapping (Figure 6.6) shows that significant excesses of native-born cases occur only in two of the inner city areas. These are the core and frame areas of the immigrant/transient district (Groups 1 and 2, Table 6.11). By contrast significantly fewer than expected native-born cases were found in the Group 13 council estates: precisely the areas where the greatest excesses of foreign-born cases were located.

CONCLUSIONS

These findings demonstrate that the ecological analysis of mental disorders should not be restricted to simple all-embracing categories. They also support the results of a previous investigation, in which the study area's first admission schizophrenics were disaggregated into marital status and family setting groups for the purposes of ecological analysis [107]. It is evident that more rigorous conceptual and methodological developments are required if ecological investigation is to prove a useful tool in the study of the incidence, spatial patterning and social-environmental precipitants of specific mental disorders among ethnic minorities and other population groups. The available evidence indicates that inter-disciplinary research probably provides the best means of investigating these complex phenomena [108-111].

Ethnic Status and Mental Illness in Urban Areas

Figure 6.6:   Distribution of Native Born Cases

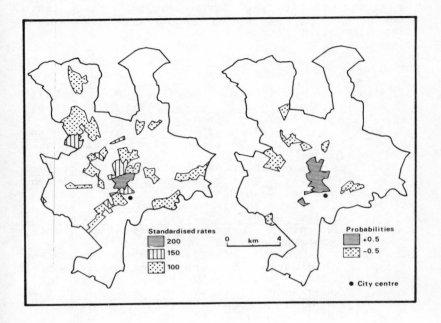

ACKNOWLEDGEMENT

The Author gratefully acknowledges that this research was funded by a grant from the Social Science Research Council.

REFERENCES

1   Cooper, B. and Morgan, H.G. (1973) Epidemiological Psychiatry, Thomas Springfield, Illinois

2. Bastide, R. (1972) The Sociology of Mental Disorder, Routledge and Kegan Paul, London

3. U.S. Bureau of the Census, Statistical Abstract of the United States, 1981, (102nd Edition) Washington, DC

4. Borrie, W.D. (1975) Population and Australia: a demographic analysis and projection, Australian Government Publishing Service, Canberra, pp. 102

5. Peach, G.C.K. (1982) "The growth and distribution of the black population in Britain 1945-1980", in D.A. Coleman (ed.) Demography of Immigrant in the United Kingdom, Academic Press, London, pp. 23-42

6. Plog, S.C. (1969) "Urbanisation, psychological disorders, and the heritages of social psychiatry", in S.C. Plog and R.B. Edgerton (eds.) Changing Perspectives in Mental Illness, Holt, Rinehart and Winston Inc., New York, pp. 288-312

7. Malzberg, B. (1969) "Are immigrants psychologically disturbed?" in S.C. Plog and R.B. Edgerton (eds.) Changing Perspectives in Mental Illness, Holt, Rinehart and Winston Inc., New York, pp 364-394

8. Gaw, A. (ed.) (1982) Cross-cultural Psychiatry, John Wright, PSG, Inc., Boston

9. Littlewood, R. and Lipsedge, M. (1982) Aliens and Alienists: Ethnic Minorities and Psychiatry, Penguin Books, Harmondsworth

10. Rack, P. (1982a) Migration and mental illness: a review of recent research in Britain, Transcultural Psychiatry Research Review, Vol. 19, pp. 151-172

11. Rack, P. (1982b) Race, Culture, and Mental Disorder, Tavistock Publications, London

12. Friessem, D.H. (1974) Psychiatric and psychosomatic diseases of foreign workers in the Federal Republic of Germany: a contribution to psychiatry of migration, Psychiatrie, Neurologie und Medinische Psycholgie, Vol. 26, pp. 78-90

13. Ramon, S., Shanin, T. and Strimpel, J. (1977) The peasant connection: Social background and mental health of migrant workers in Western Europe, Mental Health and Society, Vol. 4, pp. 270-290

14. Binder, J. and Simoes, M. (1978) Social psychiatry of migrant workers, Fortschritte to Neurologie, Psychiatrie und ihrer Grenzgebiete, Vol. 46, pp. 342-359

15. Acoss (1976) Immigrants and Mental Health: a Discussion Paper, The Australian Council of Social Service, Sydney

16. Krupinski, J. (1976) Confronting theory with data: the case of suicide, drug abuse and mental illness in Australia, The Australian and N.Z. Journal of Sociology, Vol. 12, pp. 91-100

17. Giggs, J. (1977) Mental Disorders and mental subnormality, in G.M. Howe, (ed.) A World Geography of Human Diseases, Academic Press, London, pp. 477-506

18. Stanhope, J.M. ed. (1977) Migration and Health in New Zealand and the Pacific, Epidemiology Unit, Wellington Hospital, Wellington, N.Z.

19. Burvill, P.W., Reymond J., Stampfer, H. and Carlson, J. (1982) Relation between country of birth and psychiatric admissions in Western Australia, Acta Psychiatrica Scandinavia, Vol. 66, pp. 322-335

20. Gaw, A. (1982) op. cit.

21. Littlewood, R. and Lipsedge, M. (1983) op. cit.

22. Rack, P. (1982a) op. cit.

23. Rack, P. (1982b) op. cit.

24. Jones, P.N. (1978) The distribution and diffusion of the coloured population in England and Wales, Transactions of The Institute of British Geographers, New Series Vol. 3, pp. 515-532

25. Giggs, J.A. (1979) Human health problems in urban areas, in D.T. Herbert and D.M. Smith (eds.), <u>Social Problems and the City: Geographical Perspectives</u>, Oxford University Press, Oxford, pp. 84-116
26. Smith, C.J. (1980) "Neighbourhood effects on mental health", in D.T. Herbert and R.J. Johnston (eds.) <u>Geography and the Urban environment</u>, Vol. 3, Wiley, Chichester, pp. 363-416
27. Gaw, A. (1982) op. cit.
28. Littlewood, R. and Lipsedge, M. (1982) op. cit.
29. Rack, P. (1982a) op. cit.
30. Rack, P. (1982b) op. cit.
31. Copeland, J.R.M. <u>et al</u> (1971) Differences in usage of diagnostic labels among psychiatrists in the British Isles, <u>British Journal of Psychiatry</u>, Vol. 118, pp. 629- 640
32. WHO (1973) <u>The International Pilot Study of Schizophrenia</u>, World Health Organisation, Geneva
33. Kendell, R.E. (1975) <u>The Role of Diagnosis in Psychiatry</u>, Blackwell, London.
34. Gaw, A. (1982) op. cit.
35. Littlewood, R. and Lipsedge, M. (1982) op. cit.
36. Rack, P. (1982a) op. cit.
37. Rack, P. (1982b) op. cit.
38. Littlewood and Lipsedge (1982) op. cit., p. 7
39. Smith, C. J. (1980) op. cit.
40. Giggs, J.A. (1980) Mental health and the environment, in G.M. Howe and J.A. Loraine (eds.) <u>Environmental Medicine</u>, Heinemannn Medical Books, London, pp. 281-306
41. DHSS (1977) The facilities and services of mental illness and mental handicap hospitals in England and Wales in 1976, <u>Statistical and Research Report Series, No. 10</u>, HMSO, London
42. Gaw, A. (1982) op. cit.
43. Littlewood, R. and Lipsedge, M. (1982) op. cit.
44. Rack, P. (1982a) op. cit.
45. Rack, P. (1982b) op. cit.
46. Giggs, J. (1977) op. cit.

47. Hemsi, L.K. (1967) Psychiatric mobility of West Indian immigrants: a study of first admissions in London, Social Psychiatry, Vol. 2, pp. 95-100
48. Bagley, C. (1971) Mental illness in immigrant minorities in London, Journal of Biosocial Science, Vol. 3, pp. 449-459
49. Cochrane, R. (1977) Mental illness in immigrants to England and Wales: an analysis of hospital admissions, Social Psychiatry, Vol. 12, pp. 25-35
50. Rack, P. (1982b) op. cit.
51. Faris, R.E. and Dunham, H.W. (1939) Mental Disorders in Urban Areas, University of Chicago Press, Chigaco
52. Peach, G. (1982) op. cit.
53. Peach, G.C.K. (1983) Ethnicity, in M. Pacione (ed.) Progress in Urban Geography, Croom Helm, London, pp. 103-127
54. Peach, G. (1982) op. cit.
55. Peach, G. (1982) op. cit.
56. Bastide, R. (1972) op. cit.
57. Stapleton, C. (1980) Reformulation of the family life-cycle concept: implications for residential mobility, Environment and Planning A, Vol. 12, pp. 1103-1118
58. Peach, G. (1982) op. cit.
59. Faris, R. and Dunham, H. (1939) op. cit.
60. Gaw, A. (1982) op. cit.
61. Krupinski, J. (1976) op. cit.
62. Faris, R. and Dunham, H. (1939) op. cit.
63. Schnore, L.F. (1965) The Urban Scene, Free Press, New York
64. Berry, B.J.L. (ed) (1972) City Classification Handbook: Methods and Applications, John Wiley, New York
65. Moser, C. and Scott, W. (1961) British Towns: A Statistical Study of Their Social and Economic Differences, Oliver and Boyd, Edinburgh
67. Armen, G. (1972) A classification of cities and city regions in England and Wales, 1966 Regional Studies, Vol. 6, pp. 149-182
68. US Bureau of the Census (1981) op. cit.
69. Jones, P. (1978) op. cit.

70. Giggs, J.A. (1973) The distribution of schizophrenics in Nottingham, Transactions of the Institute of British Geographers, Vol. 59, pp. 55-76

71. Taylor, S.D. (1974) "The Geography and Epidemiology of Psychiatic Disorders in Southampton", Unpublished Ph.D. thesis, University of Southampton

72. Dohrenwend, B.P. and Dohrenwend, B.S. (1974) "Psychiatric disorders in urban settings," in G. Caplan (ed.) American Handbook of Psychiatry, Vol. 2, Second Edition, Basic Books, New York, pp. 424-44

73. Dear, M. (1977) Psychiatric patients and the inner city, Annals of the Association of American Geographers, Vol. 67, pp. 588-594

74. Sainsbury, P. (1955) Suicide in London, Maudsley Monograph No. 1., Chapman and Hall, London

75. Dever, G.E.A. (1972) 'Leukaemia and housing: an intra-urban analysis', in N.D. McGlashan, (ed.) Medical Geography: Techniques and Field Studies, Methuen, London, pp. 233-245

76. Boal, F.W. (1976) "Ethnic residential segregation", in D.T. Herbert and R.J. Johnston, (eds.) Social Areas in Cities, Wiley, London, pp. 57-95

77. Giggs, J. (1979) op. cit.

78. Faris, R. and Dunham, H. (1939) op. cit.

79. Knox, P. (1982) Urban Social Geography, Longman, London

80. Peach, G. (1982) op. cit.

81. Peach, G. (1983) op. cit.

82. Boal, F. (1976) op. cit.

83. Hall, P., Thomas, R., Gracey, H., and Drewett, R. (1973) Megalopolis Denied: The Containment of Urban England, 1945-1979, Vol. 1., Allen and Unwin, London

84. Giggs, J.A. (1970) Fringe expansion and suburbanisation around Nottingham: a metropolitan area approach, East Midland Geographer, Vol. 1, pp. 9-18

85. Jones, P. N. (1978) op. cit.

86. Giggs, J.A. (1973) High rates of schizophrenia among immigrants in Nottingham, Nursing Times, Sept. 20, pp. 1210-1212

87. Wing, J.K.   (1972)   Epidemiology of
     Schizophrenia, British Journal of Hospital
     Medicine, Vol. 8, pp. 364-368
88. Littlewood, R. and Lipsedge, M. (1982) op.
     cit.
89. Littlewood,   R.   and   Lipsedge,   M.   (1978)
     Migration, ethnicity and diagnosis,
     Psychiatrica   Clinica,   Vol.   11, pp.
     15-22
90. Peach, G. (1982) op. cit.
91. Peach, G. (1982) op. cit.
92. Boal, F. (1976) op. cit.
93. Jones, P.N.   (1979) Ethnic Areas in British
     Cities, in D.T. Herbert and D.M. Smith
     (eds.)   Social   Problems and the City:
     Geographical   Perspectives,   Oxford
     University Press, Oxford, pp. 158-185
94. Giggs, J. (1979) op. cit.
95. Smith, C.J. (1980) op. cit.
96. Faris, R. and Dunham, H. (1939) op. cit.
97. Levy, L. and Rowitz, L. (1973) The Ecology
     of   Mental   Disorder,   Behavioural
     Publications, New York
98. Hare, E.H. (1956) Family Setting and the Urban
     Distribution of Schizophrenia, Journal of
     Mental Science, Vol. 102, pp. 753-760
99. Ibid., pp. 755
100. Giggs,   J.A.   and   Mather,   P.M.   (1983)
     Contemporary   Perspectives   on   the
     Geography of Mental Illness in Urban
     Areas,   Report   series   on   Applied
     Geography,   No.   3,   Department of
     Geography,   Nottingham   University,
     Nottingham
101. Lawrence, D. (1974) Black Migrants: White
     Natives,   Cambridge University Press,
     London
102. Husain,   M.S.   (1975)   The   increase and
     distribution   of   New   Commonwealth
     immigrants in Greater Nottingham, The
     East Midland Geographer, Vol. 6, pp. 105-
     129
103. Simpson,   A.   (1981)   Stacking the Decks,
     Nottingham   and   District   Community
     Relations Council, Nottingham
104. Norcliffe, G.B. (1977) Inferential Statistics
     for Geographers, Hutchinson, London
105. Faris, R. and Dunham, H. (1939) op. cit.
106. Levy, L. and Rowitz, L. (1973) op. cit.

107. Giggs, J.A. (1983) Schizophrenia and ecological structure in Nottingham, in J. Blunden and N.D. McGlashan, (eds) Geographical Aspects of Health, Academic Press, London

108. Sainsbury, P. (1972) The Social Relations of Suicide. The value of a combined epidemiological and case study approach, Social Science and Medicine, Vol. 6, pp. 189-198

109. Bagley, C. and Jacobson, S. (1976) Ecological variation of three types of Suicide, Psychological Medicine, No. 6, pp. 423-427.

110. Bagley, C., Jacobson, S. and Rehin, A. (1976) Completed suicide: a taxonomic analysis of clinical and social data, Psychological Medicine, Vol. 6, pp. 429-438

111. Jacobson, S., Bagley, C., and Rehin, A. (1976) Clinical and social variables which differentiate suicide, open and accident verdicts, Psychological Medicine, Vol. 6, pp. 417-421

Chapter 7

HEALTH CARE AND ETHNIC MINORITIES IN DENMARK

Marianne Lauridsen

INTRODUCTION

The issue of ethnic minorities in Denmark is a
relatively new phenomenon. For centuries Denmark
was a country with a very homogeneous population,
even though it was the destination of some migrants.
These early migrants were in many cases refugees
from countries not notably different from Denmark,
compared to the countries from which it has received
new inhabitants within the last few decades. Being
refugees these former migrants came in relatively
small numbers and, knowing it would be impossible
for them to return to their country of origin, they
had in general a strong wish to become integrated or
even assimilated into Danish society.
        It was not until the late 1960s and the
beginning of the 1970s that in-migration on a
considerable scale occurred. Migration in the
context used here is synonymous with a flow of
foreign workers, which in the case of Denmark came
mainly from Yugoslavia, Turkey and Pakistan, but
also included Arabs, mainly from North Africa. This
migration to Denmark was encouraged and supported by
Danish Society, in the sense that there was a demand
for manpower, to which the migrants responded,
because of the prosperity at that period. The
migrants that arrived in the first place were mainly
males who came with the intention of working in the
country for a few years in order to save money with
which they could return to their country of origin
and start a new life with resources to draw on.
Therefore, the migrants who came to Denmark at that
time, generally speaking, saw no purpose in becoming
integrated into Danish society, and Danish society
saw no need in trying very hard to ensure their
integration.
        During the first years of immigration to
Denmark problems were relatively few. In the labour
market vacancies were abundant, including jobs which

did not require high technical skills or great knowledge of Danish, and therefore such jobs could quite easily be undertaken by newly arrived migrant workers. As these migrant workers rarely brought their families with them there were few problems related to health care, social security and education, as demands on these social services were initially low.

However, the oil crisis in the middle 1970s precipitated a period of economic decline and, as a consequence, the need for manpower diminished. Since the migrant workers were generally unskilled or at least less skilled than their Danish colleagues, they suffered most heavily from loss of employment as a consequence of the economic recession.

The Danish Government foreseeing such problems, imposed in 1973 a ban on immigration from developing countries, but endorsed a policy of allowing the family of a migrant worker currently resident in Denmark to join him. This policy, combined with the fact that the recession was world-wide and consequently the motivation for return migration was not very strong, has through the years actually resulted in an increased number of migrants to Denmark.

It was not until the late 1970s that Danish Society realised that its 'laissez-faire' policy towards immigrants and migrant workers was no longer appropriate and that there now was a need for formulating a policy concerning ethnic minorities. This paper begins with a brief description of the ethnic groups in Denmark, the Danish political system and health network and how they have responded to the issue of formulating a general policy regarding ethnic minorities. This is then followed by a discussion of the health care problems of the ethnic minorities and how they are being tackled. The paper concludes with an assessment of the degree of success achieved.

THE ETHNIC GROUPS IN DENMARK

In Denmark 'foreigners' are defined as people without Danish citizenship, who have stayed in Denmark for more than three months. The total population of the country is approximately 5,000,000 people, of whom some 104,000 are migrants according to the above definition. Of the total number of migrants, 104,000 (about 2% of the total population), just under one-half (51,000) consists of people who came from either the Nordic countries (especially Norway and Sweden) the countries of the European Economic Community or North-America. The rest - a little more than half of the foreign part of population, or approximately 53,000 people - came from the so-called developing countries. Among these, Turkey, Yugoslavia and Pakistan are predominant, accounting for some 16,800, 7,400 and 6,700 nationals respectively living in Denmark [1].

Throughout the last decade the 'foreigner' element of the Danish population has increased by nearly 10%. The number of foreigners coming from the Nordic countries, the EEC and North America declined over this period but this has been offset by an increase in the population from developing countries. At first glance this increase may seem strange given that Denmark had imposed a ban on immigration from the developing countries. The increase can be partly explained by the policy of accepting the families of previous migrants and partly a consequence of the higher fertility-rate common to these groups when compared to the indigenous population.

To summarise Danish migration policy is directed towards some 1% of the total population, which suggests when judged by international standards that the migrant issue in Denmark is not of a comparative size. Even though this may be the case it was felt that there was a need to formulate a general migration policy in order to facilitate the integration of migrants into Danish society.

THE POLITICAL-ADMINISTRATIVE SYSTEM IN DENMARK

Since 1970, when a reform of the structure for governing Denmark was carried out, the country has had the following three political-administrative levels:

- state
- county
- municipality

The key objective of the reform was decentralisation based on appropriate units; that is problems should be solved at the 'lowest' possible, but sufficient and secure, level. Administratively and politically the country was divided into 14 counties (averaging 300,000 inhabitants) and 275 municipalities (which vary from 5,000 and 250,000 inhabitants). The political-administrative reform was followed by an economic reform of block-grants, in order to, among other things, facilitate the process of organising local services according to local needs. This structure of government and decision-making is discussed further through the example of the health care system in Denmark.

THE DANISH HEALTH SYSTEM [2]

There is no Ministry of Health in Denmark. Responsibility for health is spread amongst several ministries as Table 7.1 indicates, with the Ministry of the Interior undertaking the majority of the functions specific to the provision of health care.

State or Central Level

The Ministry of the Interior has the overall responsibility for the health care system; that is, legislation and planning concerning hospitals, national health insurance, primary health care, public health schemes, drugs, health professionals, including post-graduate training of doctors and dentists (and a few other groups of health professionals), as well as education of non-academic health professionals. Within the structure of the Ministry of the Interior there is also the National Council of Prevention. The Council has been assigned the task of undertaking a critical evaluation of the existing measures to promote health within and outside the health sector, and of presenting proposals to further preventive efforts in all sectors, which may, in one way or another, imply effects injurious to health.

The Ministry of Education was until recently responsible for undergraduate education of academic health professionals only, as well as for the State University Hospital in Copenhagen, the only remaining state-owned hospital. However as from the first of January, 1984, the responsibility for undergraduate education of non-academic health professionals was transferred to the Ministry of Education, whilst the Ministry of the Interior assumed responsibility for the State University Hospital in Copenhagen. This change will have no implication for post-graduate training of health professionals as this responsibility continues to reside with the Ministry of the Interior.

Health Care and Ethnic Minorities in Denmark

Table 7.1: Danish Health System (State Level)

Ministries	Areas of Responsibility
Finance	- national economy - economic planning - negotiate state-wages
Interior	- legislative, advisory, approving and supervisory on (primary care) - public health insurance - personal preventive services - Copenhagen University Hospital - postgraduate medical training - postgraduate training of health personnel - preventive council
Social affairs	- social assistance and counselling - nursing homes and planning
Education	- medical education - training of health personnel
Environmental Affairs	- environmental hygiene - food safety
Labour	- occupational health services
National Board of Health	- advises all ministries on health issues

Source: Public Administration and Health Care in
Denmark.   (Reproduced with permission)

     At the central level, the National Board of
Health has an advisory function not only to all
ministries, but also to health authorities at lower
levels.

County Level
The counties have the responsibility for managing
the hospitals and for financing primary health care
through the national health insurance system (Figure
7.1).   It should be mentioned, that primary health
care in Denmark is based on agreements between the
Associations of the Health Professionals and the

Health Care and Ethnic Minorities in Denmark

Figure 7.1:   Danish Health System (county level)

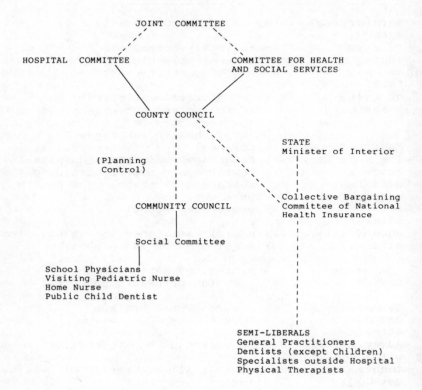

Source: Public Administration and Health Care in Denmark
           (Reproduced with permission)

Association of County Councils. Therefore, in principle, general practitioners and dentists are not employees, but they do have to perform their services according to the criteria laid down in the agreements.

The counties also have responsibility for education of non-academic health professionals, such as nurses and assistant nurses. This is due to the fact, that their education contains a large element of practical training, which usually takes place in hospital.

Municipal Level

The municipalities are responsible for public health schemes which include, among others, children's dental care, school physicians, and home visiting nurses. The municipalities are responsible as well for the adjoining social sector, which is important considering that social conditions may sometimes underlie certain symptoms of a health related nature.

DANISH HEALTH POLICY

Denmark, like many other industrialised countries, has adopted a general health policy characterised by stressing the importance of preventive measures. Advanced skills of health professionals combined with the seemingly endless sophistication of new technologies have made tremendous strides in developing highly specialised treatment for illness and disease but such improvements are costly to effect, and therefore unlikely to have other than a limited impact on the general level of health of the population. Since such sophisticated forms of health care can only benefit a small number it seems prudent for any health policy to emphasise the advantages of prevention in order to try to minimise the necessity for such sophisticated treatment. The rationale for greater emphasis on preventive measures was one which sought to meet existing demands in the health sector whilst, at the same time, attempting to constrain the level of expenditure.

The policy emphasises the need for a change in perspective within the health care sector in the hope that such a change will lead to better utilisation of the limited resources available.

Health Care and Ethnic Minorities in Denmark

Primary health care is being favoured at the expense
of hospital care, and within the hospitals day-care
and open wards are preferred at the expense of
traditional hospitalisation. Within the public
health schemes demands for routine examinations have
been reduced in favour of examinations according to
accepted needs. This is particularly important
when talking about ethnic minorities, and their
particular needs and use of the health care system.
However, before discussing the health needs of
Denmark's ethnic minorities, a brief description of
the country's migration policy seems in order.

THE POLITICAL-ADMINISTRATIVE STRUCTURE FOR MIGRANT
ISSUES

The Minister of the Interior has overall
responsibility for the co-ordination of Denmark's
migration policy. It is however important to
emphasise that responsibility for activities within
the different sectors or ministries remains with the
minister responsible. A government committee has
been appointed, consisting of the seven most
relevant ministries (Interior, Education, Social
Affairs, Justice, Labour, Cultural Affairs and
Housing) to liaise with and to provide the necessary
support for the Ministry of the Interior to enable
it to discharge its overall responsibility in this
area of government policy. To support the
ministries in their work, a committee of officers
from the afore-mentioned ministries has been
appointed. This committee is responsible for
preparing meetings of the ministerial committee
including preparations of proposals for new
activities, and is, of course, responsible for
carrying out decisions taken by the committee of
ministers.
    There also exists a specific committee for
contact between state and municipal levels which is
co-ordinated by the Ministry of the Interior. This
Committee was established in acknowledgement of the
fact that the municipality is the level where
contact between migrants and different authorities
takes place, and, consequently, it is the level
where problems are presented and action demanded.
For the Central administration, it is of great
importance to receive information about 'where the
shoe pinches', but it is of value, as well, to
discuss considerations on new initiatives with those
who wear the shoes.

A very important - if not the most important - element in Danish migration policy is the desire for active participation from the migrants themselves. To create a forum through which such participation could be channelled an advisory committee (the Council of Migrants) has been established. The Council is chaired by a civil servant from the Ministry of the Interior and consists at present of representatives from 20 ethnic organisations. Besides being a forum for exchanges of views the Council has an advisory function to the government and the central and state administrations, insofar as the Council should be granted an opportunity to give an opinion on proposals of all kinds relevant to the migrants and their life-conditions. The Council of Migrants has of course the opportunity as well of putting forward its own proposals.

The Council, when originally established, consisted of one representative from each of the migrant societies which receives financial support from the Ministry of the Interior. This representation was, however, not without certain drawbacks and could be criticised on a number of grounds but a start had to be made somewhere, in order to ensure that the administrative and consultative structure was capable of meeting its early objectives.

Nonetheless, the early days proved to be a learning experience for both parties. On the government's side, much was learnt about each migrant society and their basic rules and regulations. As for the societies themselves, to qualify for financial support, they were required to demonstrate that they had a 'democratic structure' - an elected board or state of officers - and that their affairs were managed according to standard economic principles.

It must be acknowledged, however, that it was more or less accidental whether or not a society of migrants was aware of the possibility of getting financial support and thus able to become a member of the Council. Membership of 'organised' migrants also varied very much from nationality to nationality, mainly due to the different traditions they have brought with them to Denmark. Therefore the representativeness of the Council could and can be called to question.

Given these so-called 'teething' problems and although its initial working experience has generally been very positive, the Council was nonetheless given the task of putting forward proposals for its re-organisation. On the basis mainly of discussion in the Council, but also from soundings taken at a meeting with representatives from all known societies of migrants, it was decided that in the future membership of the Council should be by direct election. The first direct election of the 'new' council is scheduled to take place just after Christmas 1984.

GENERAL MIGRATION POLICY IN DENMARK

The formulation of a policy for immigrants is a relatively new phenomenon in Denmark and the issue has been debated a number of times in Parliament within the past four years. The main objective of the general policy has been defined as integration of the ethnic groups in question into Danish society with due respect to their cultural and social background. One cannot emphasise too strongly the fact that in Denmark the focus is on integration and not assimilation. The core of the migration policy is that the migrants in the long run shall be able to function in Danish society on an equal footing with the Danes, and therefore there is absolutely no purpose in trying to transform them into Danes. In fact, the government financially supports the activities which take place within the framework of the various societies of migrants, and which are aimed largely at preserving their cultural heritage. In the general policy it is further acknowledged that, basically, integration is the responsibility of the individual, but, of course, society has to establish supportive measures in order to facilitate the process of integration [3]. Another element in the policy could be described as 'the necessity of acceptance of cultural losses'. Moving from one country to another does mean that one loses part of one's identity - both literally and in a figurative sense - and that one has to give up certain values. Part of the Danish policy is founded on the belief that the migrants must accept this. To a certain extent they must accept the values and standards of Danish society, not because these values and standards are better than those in their countries of origin, but because these are the ones of the society in which the migrants currently live. Equally the Danes have to accept that in certain areas the migrants prefer - and should have the right - to live according to values of life which may be different from those of the Danes. In other words, in applying the policy on migrants it is important to keep a balance in particular between what one is demanding of the migrants and what one is demanding of Danes.

It will be recalled that the key feature of the Danish migration policy is integration. The following are illustrative of three of the means identified for reaching this objective. First there is the teaching of Danish; secondly a necessary supporting system, within the health and social sector and the labour market; and, thirdly, a sensible policy concerning housing. Within these sectors different initiatives have been taken in order to facilitate the possibilities of achieving the objective of integration. Apart from the health and social sector, these initiatives will not be described in great detail, instead a brief outline is given.

All migrants are encouraged to take basic courses in Danish, courses that are free of charge. Not only the (male) workers, but also the women as well. For the workers a basic knowledge of Danish is often vital but for the women it can be a means of breaking any isolation they may feel. A feeling that may even influence their family life in view of the fact that children rather quickly – when entering school – get to learn Danish.

As unemployment rates are higher among migrants than among Danes special programmes have been introduced on the labour-market which are aimed at the improvement of their professional skills (combined with teaching the specialised Danish vocabulary, which is necessary for carrying out a specific job). Special efforts are likewise being made to help young migrants and female migrants, who often have even greater problems than male migrants in entering the labour-market.

With respect to housing it is a commonplace that migrants often settle in the same small areas. There is a feeling however that this may influence the integration process in a negative way, probably due to more or less psychological factors. Consequently a committee has been established with among others a representative appointed by the Council of Migrants to analyse this and to make proposals for overcoming these problems.

In general, however, since resources are limited the policy has been based on the principle of 'accepted needs', and by this it is assumed that people from developing countries are in greatest need of supportive measures. The rationale for such an approach is partly because they have their origin in countries which differ fundamentally from Denmark, economically, socially and culturally, and partly because they do not benefit, generally speaking, from mutual agreements concerning for example legal rights, and social security as do people from the Nordic countries and EEC.

HEALTH CARE AND ETHNIC MINORITIES

The theme 'Health Care and Ethnic Minorities' can, of course, be understood in different ways, depending upon one's chosen viewpoint. Looking at it from an administrative perspective first, thoughts will be about the actual provision of health care for these groups and in particular consideration will be given as to whether or not one should provide a service according to the specific needs of ethnic minorities. To answer this question it is necessary to be able to identify these specific needs, and this can be done through statistics and through research of different kinds. Given that the question of migration policy is a rather new phenemenon in Denmark, the statistics as well as research concerning migrants could be said still to be in a somewhat preliminary phase, or at any rate not fully developed.

In Denmark, there is not a special research institute which has been assigned the task of conducting research on or about ethnic minorities but, despite this, different intitiatives have been taken, of which the following are illustrations. The Ministry of the Interior did propose to inititiate a broad study on the life-conditions of migrants living in Denmark, a study which was to be conducted by the Danish National Institute of Social Research. The Institute in the past has undertaken similar studies on the total population and it seems sensible to include ethnic minorities in such a survey since the two studies would have formed a good basis for comparison. Unfortunately it was not possible to obtain the necessary funding, and so a less ambitious study was proposed.

The Institute is now engaged on a study on the life-conditions of migrants based only on information which can be drawn from existing statistical sources (data-banks for example). Therefore the study will not include personal interviews with members of the different ethnic communities, but hopefully the use of routinely gathered statistical data will uncover areas which ought to be studied in greater depth.

Another initiative has been taken by the Danish Social Science Research Council which has decided to give research concerning migrant issues high priority in the period 1984-1987 [4]. Within this time frame several projects have been initiated or proposed by individual researchers as well as by institutes of different kinds. Some of these projects but by no means all are specifically concentrating on health issues.

Mention should also be made of the initiative which Denmark, Norway and Sweden, under the auspices of the Nordic Council of Ministers, have started, which is a joint-venture project on 'the migrants and the local health and social services'. Since there are many similarities in the migration policy of all three countries but also some differences in the way in which each of them have structured their health and social services, the results of this project are anticipated with great interest.

Lastly it should not be forgotten that at the local level several initiatives have been taken as well which generally focus on the life-conditions of the migrants living in the local community. Many of those municipalities which have relatively large numbers of migrants have prepared reports on the implications for the local community of the settlement of 'foreigners', including implications for the local health care service (primary health care). While such initiatives to try to understand the ethnic individual are both welcome and necessary it will be some time before any change or benefit is forthcoming. In the meantime, the different ethnic groups in Denmark do have some real and particular problems which demand early intervention.

The different cultural and linguistic backgrounds of the migrants (as patients) and the health professionals do cause problems which inevitably lead to poorer quality treatment for ethnic than indigenous groups. Some examples of the problems relating to linguistic differences are:

- the migrants as patients have difficulties in explaining their problems;
- the health professionals have difficulty in understanding the problem as it is presented;

- the migrants as patients have difficulties in understanding the 'message' given to them by the health professional.

Examples of the problems related to cultural differences usually cited are:

- the health professionals' difficulty in understanding the patients' real problem, which often may be of a psychosomatic nature, and related in part to alienation within Danish society;
- the attitude among some ethnic groups as regards the conception of the body and how it functions (many subjects may be more or less taboo);
- the attitude towards preventive measures among many ethnic groups - a fundamental factor in the Danish health care system - is far from being sufficiently developed.

These problems have had their consequences, in that one can now find many children of ethnic groups with serious deficiency diseases (such as anaemia and rickets), which were previously almost eradicated in Denmark and certainly amongst the host population. One can also find ethnic minority women with serious abdominal diseases, which have not been treated properly in due time partly because most health professionals are not used to diagnosing such diseases. To this already complicated picture one can add health problems (such as respiratory diseases and bronchitis) which are often associated with or related to inadequate housing [5].

The over-riding principle of the Danish health care system in responding to the specific needs of the ethnic groups is that there should be no differentiation between groups in the sense that there are different services for different groups. In other words the operative philosophy is one which assumes that the structural mechanisms for health care are adequate and therefore what is required is a better understanding by those working within the system of the particular requirements of ethnic patients. To this end efforts have been concentrated on establishing supporting measures within the existing health care system. Some examples of these measures are:

- improvement of interpreting facilities
  (necessary interpretation can, under the
  National Health Insurance, be obtained by the
  general practitioner free of charge for the
  patient);
- provision of information/material prepared
  in a short and concise manner. This method of
  spreading information does however have its
  limitations, due to problems of illiteracy
  plus the fact that some of the spoken
  languages (dialects) do not have a written
  form;
- material consisting mainly of pictures may
  be a way to overcoming this problem, but it
  should be borne in mind that some subjects
  may be more or less taboo when presented
  figuratively;
- tape-recorded information has been used both
  in primary health care and in hospitals with
  satisfactory results.

The above-mentioned initiatives are all aimed
primarily at overcoming linguistic and communication
problems, but as has already been indicated problems
caused by differences in cultural background may be
of even greater importance and consequently may
cause even greater problems.

Information is one of the keys in the efforts
to overcome many of these problems. Not only
information for the migrants, but - equally as
important if not more important - information for
health professionals about the values and standards
of life of the migrants and their countries of
origin, which may lead to a better understanding
among health professionals about the way in which
migrants react or could be expected to react in
certain situations. A close ally of improved
information for both migrants and health
professionals is a programme of post-graduate and/or
post-experience training for health professionals
also as a means to improving their awareness of the
different health needs of the ethnic minorities.

The establishment of local groups of migrant
women has proved to be a very good way of breaking
down some of the barriers contributing to their
isolation and, at the same time, has been a good way
of spreading information about public health schemes
for children, public health schemes for care during
pregnancy, and health promotion in general. Such
groups are often managed by peripatetic paediatric
nurses, and meeting places are situated very close
to the migrants home (a meeting-place, for

example, could be an unoccupied apartment in an apartment building) in order to facilitate the participation and to overcome possible objections to the idea of migrant women receiving 'out-reach' activities. It is worth stressing once again that in all the different health care schemes and in health care services in general, high priority has been given to the provision of services according to ostensible needs, and not to the provision of care according to more or less fixed standards. With this in mind it has been the policy that migrants, especially women and children, generally speaking, are persons having <u>a priori</u> accepted needs for special attendance.

CONCLUSIONS

The main elements of Danish migration policy, including provision of health care for the ethnic minorities, could be summarised in the following way. The objective of the policy is that of integration with due respect given to the migrants cultural and linguistic background. The success of this integration policy is dependent, of course, on the migrants themselves as well as on the Danes. They are expected to assume part of the responsibility for their health just as the Danes must assume the responsibility for providing the necessary financial measures and support which will facilitate the process. It is therefore essential to keep a balance between what Danish society demands of them and what Danish society demands of itself.

At State level the necessary active co-operation is channelled through the Council of Migrants which through the new elective procedure should ensure that it will become the forum for reflecting the opinions representative of the migrants living in Denmark. This in turn should provide the mechanism by which the local level can initiate and implement appropriate practical programmes for ethnic minorities.

The provision of health care for ethnic minorities presents a set of new challenges for Denmark but ones it is believed should be solved within the existing structure of the Danish health care system by provision of supporting measures: such as better information - both for health professionals as well as for the migrants themselves; post-graduate training of health professionals; and a programme of community based case-work. The problems are self-evidently not easy to solve, but if everybody involved takes an active part and tries to look at the problems as a challenge rather than an obstacle to be repressed, it will be possible to build a better society for all.

REFERENCES

1. Indenrigsministeriat: Statistik om Indvandrene (1983)
    (The Ministry of the Interior, Statistics concerning migrants, 1983.)
2. National Board of Health (1984) Public Administration and Health Care in Denmark, National Board of Health, Copenhagen
3. Redegorelse   i   folketinget om indvandrerpolitikken den 12 april 1984 af indenrigsministeren
    Folketingstidende 1983, spalte 8978-8989
    (Statement in Parliament of Migration Policy (12 April, 1983) by the Minister of the Interior)
    Official report of parliamentary proceedings, 1983, column 8978-8989
4. Statens Samfundsvidenskabelige Forskningsrad: Indvandrerforskning i Danmark, 1983
    (Danish Social Science Research Council: Research in Denmark concerning Ethnic minorities, 1983.)
5. Donovan, J. (1984) Ethnicity and health: a research review, Social Science and Medicine, Vol. 19, pp. 663-670

Chapter 8

INNER CITY RESIDENTS, ETHNIC MINORITIES AND
PRIMARY HEALTH CARE IN THE WEST MIDLANDS

Mark Johnson

INTRODUCTION

The presence of ethnic minorities in the larger
cities of Britain is not an especially new feature
of our society. Consequently it must be assumed
that the British medical profession has been dealing
with black clients as patients for as long as it has
existed as a scientific discipline. However, it is
observable that as suggested in chapter 1 the
majority of references in medical publishing which
deal with this issue have discussed it in terms of
an 'immigrant problem', implying that the special
needs of black people represented a passing
phase [1]. Early publications for the medical
profession were in the vein of 'Port Medicine' [2],
concentrating on exotic diseases and issues of
public health, and rarely regarded seriously the
problems of immigrant groups in terms of social and
economic disadvantage.

Subsequent developments in medical awareness
began to show a greater understanding of the needs
of ethnic minority patients. In particular,
clinical researchers became interested in specific
diseases such as sickle-cell anaemia [3] or
osteomalacia/rickets [4] which were largely to be
found among members of more narrowly defined
minorities. Practitioners were also becoming more
aware of their own needs to understand the 'culture'
of black patients, both for clinical and
administrative reasons. This has led to a number
of articles and booklets [5,6] seeking to inform the
doctor or nurse about the varieties of Asian culture
in particular. Pressure has also been growing from
client-orientated groups [7-9] for a more radical
review of service provision. At the same time the
National Health Service (NHS), under pressure from
reorganisation and resource cuts (or re-allocation)
was beginning to review critically the provision of
health services in the inner city [10,11]. This has

provided an opportunity to rethink the profession's attitude towards service provision for ethnic minority groups, but regrettably there is a distinct lack of information for policy makers about the interface between the community and the service [12].

With notable exceptions [13-15], very few researchers appear to have considered the quality of care provided to minority clients and not infrequently studies of the 'quality of care' provided to minority clients in inner city areas have appeared to lack any comprehension of the 'race issue' except perhaps to refer to the proportions of overseas-qualified doctors [16]. This issue has been addressed in some detail in chapter 4. Alternatively, studies have focused upon problems associated with ethnic minorities in a manner likely to 'blame the victims' for poor uptake of services [17] or by concentrating on the provision of interpreting services [18]. Such interpreters as exist in the NHS tend to be hospital-based although certain health centres in Birmingham have employed them (using Inner City Partnership funds), and recourse is frequently made to the skills of ancillary staff who are often not trained either in medicine or interpreting. Rarely is the 'overseas doctor' (usually Asian) seen as contributing to the solution although, as will be demonstrated that is the answer found by many Asian patients. (The desirability of this, of course, in terms of the range of choice for patients or in making the assumption that Asian doctors share a common culture with Asian patients, is a matter that is wide open for debate.) Given existing demographic trends (but not assuming that Britain's inner cities will become entirely black ghettos) and the known inequalities in our society that affect ethnic minorities, there is a pressing need for studies which take seriously the question of delivery of services to this group. This study, built on a larger enquiry into the use and provison of 'public goods' (welfare services) in the West Midlands, attempts to examine some of the key questions relating to under- and over-utilisation of primary health care and to combat the myths which appear to have developed about the position of ethnic minorities, frequently characterised as 'immigrants', in relation to the NHS.

METHODS

A survey of over 2,000 households in selected wards of Birmingham, Coventry and Wolverhampton containing substantial proportions of ethnic minority populations was carried out in 1981 to establish ethnic variations in service use and receipt, including data on primary health service provision [19]. Households were identified using standard stratified random sampling techniques and a simple randomised screening procedure. Response rates in excess of 80% were achieved and the population confirmed as representative by reference to 1981 Census data. Information was obtained from the head of household or spouse by a trained interviewer, and an attempt made to obtain roughly equal numbers of male and female respondents (except in single-adult households). The survey was concerned in particular to examine whether ethnic minority clients made excessive or unjustified demands upon the health service. In order to compare like with like, however, the survey dealt only with households containing people under the age of 60 - and while a third or more of inner city white residents are over this age, elderly ethnic minority residents are rare. Their problems have been addressed by a recent specific survey [20]. Data here are presented categorised by 'ethnic group' based upon respondent self-assessment but confirmed by interviewer observation.

REGISTRATION

Contrary to expectations, 99% of all groups (white, Asian and Afro-Caribbean) were registered with an NHS General Practitioner (GP), and only about 10% were not reportedly registered with one practising in their immediate area of residence, although there were some variations between the survey wards (Table 8.1). Asians were most likely to be locally registered, and two-thirds were registered with a GP of Asian origin, a further 10% being registered with practices containing an Asian doctor (Table 8.2). One in four of the whites in the survey was also registered either with an Asian doctor or a 'mixed' practice, as were more than one in three Afro-Caribbeans. Of the 171 practices identified, 59 were Asian and 21 'mixed'. It was notable that where more 'mixed' practices were to be found, white

Table 8.1: GP Registration and Consultation Rates
in Previous Year (Percentage)

	White	Asian	Afro Caribbean
Locally Registered	88	96	89
Registered Elsewhere	11	4	10
Not Registered	1	-	(2)[a]
	100%	100%	
(N)	(915)	(867)	(365)

[a] Under 2% numbers rounded.

$x^2 = 49.0$ sig p< 0.001
  df = 4

	White	Asian	Afro Caribbean
No. Visits in Year	32	13	23
One/two in year	35	21	31
3-5 in year	15	24	21
6 or more in year	18	24	21
Not Known	-	18	4
	100%	100%	100%
(N)	(915)	(867)	(365)

$x^2 = 305.8$ Sig p<0.001
df = 8

Table 8.2: Ethnicity of General Practice with
which Registered

Doctors	Ethnicity of Respondent		
	White	Asian	Afro-Caribbean
All White	75%	25%	61%
Mixed	15%	10%	99%
All Asian	9%	66%	29%
	100%	100%	100%
(N)	(850)	(820)	(340)

x^2 = 587.7 Sig p<0.001
    df = 4

Number of Practices

White	83	54	62
Mixed	20	11	8
Asian	31	46	26

x^2 = 22.5 Sig p<0.001
df = 4

respondents' suspicion of 'foreign doctors' was
least! On closer examination it appeared that there
were some spatial patterns suggesting that ethnic
groups did not always occupy the same socio-spatial
territory.

It may be self-evident that the location of a
person's GP in relation to his/her residence is
important in affecting access, but it is nonetheless
an underdocumented field of research [21]. The
contention is that the concentration of ethnic
minorities in inner city areas has effects upon the
services they are able to receive, and on the degree
of choice they can exercise. Equally, when
'dispersed' in more suburban areas they can suffer
from the lack of 'appropriate' and sensitive
services, or direct racism. Anecdotally,
researchers may become aware that some practitioners

resist registration by black patients, and it is consistently reported in the medical press that at least some inner-city GPs provide a less than satisfactory standard of care. In the light of this it is of interest to examine the data from the survey as it relates to registration, both as perceived by patient/respondents, and as observed by locating doctors' surgeries.

Subjective assessments of doctors' nearness, however, are notoriously unreliable: roughly half of all white and Afro-Caribbean respondents said their GP was 'the nearest' while nearly two-thirds (62%) of Asians believed theirs was, and one in ten (11%) said they were 'all about the same'. Consideration of the objective facts illustrated in Figures 8.1-8.4 would not support this belief. That said, comment cannot be made about the quality of care received in any 'objective' fashion although it was observed that inner-city residents generally seemed more likely to have been seen by their own GP on a night visit rather than by a 'deputising service', especially if that GP was apparently of Asian origin. This at least might be seen to be a 'good thing' by many patients.

There is, in the areas covered by the survey, no shortage of GPs (Table 8.2, part 2) although there are no data on their 'list sizes' or any other information on the quality of care they can supply. However, it is apparent from Table 8.3 that there was not an equivalent likelihood of being registered with a GP within 'walking distance' of home. Curiously, the results are far from consistent and must reflect the outcome of a process of 'supply and demand'. The Afro-Caribbean respondents, overall, seem most unlikely to be registered with a very local practice but to have their doctor 'elsewhere in the inner city'. The exception is Wolverhampton (Figure 8.1), where Asians are extremely unlikely to have a local GP and much more likely to be registered in Blakenhall or Whitmore Reans, two other 'inner city' areas. Whites and Afro-Caribbeans were more likely to go to surgeries further out of town. In Coventry, by contrast, very few Asians were registered outside the 'Railway Triangle' that marks the major area of Asian settlement in the city (Figure 8.2). Indeed, this may explain part of the discrepancy demonstrated by the table, where it can be observed that in Selly Oak there are only slight differences between white

Figure 8.1: Location and Usage of Doctors in South West Wolverhampton

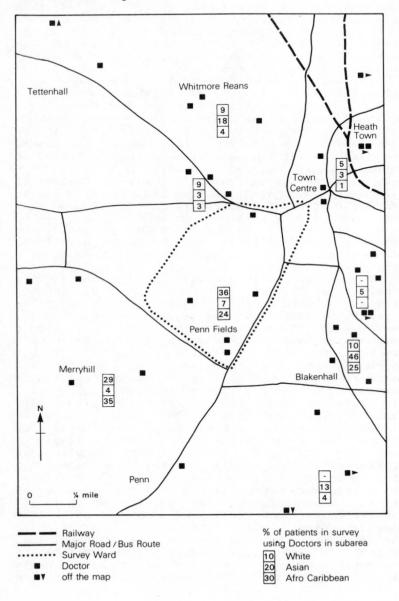

Tettenhall

Whitmore Reans

| 9 |
| 18 |
| 4 |

Heath Town

Town Centre

| 5 |
| 3 |
| 1 |

| 9 |
| 3 |
| 3 |

| - |
5

| 36 |
| 7 |
| 24 |

Penn Fields

| 10 |
| 46 |
| 25 |

Blakenhall

Merryhill

| 29 |
| 4 |
| 35 |

N

Penn

0   ¼ mile

| - |
| 13 |
| 4 |

Railway
Major Road / Bus Route
Survey Ward
Doctor
off the map

% of patients in survey
using Doctors in subarea

10	White
20	Asian
30	Afro Caribbean

Figure 8.2: Location and Usage of Doctors in North Coventry

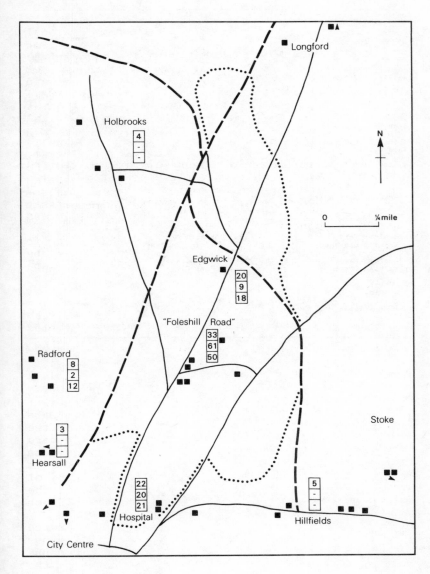

Ethnic Minorities and Primary Health Care

Table 8.3: Nearness to GP with whom Registered

Inner City Sample (%)

	Wolverhampton			Birmingham			Coventry		
	White	Asian	A/C[a]	White	Asian	A/C	White	Asian	A/C
In Same Ward (Walking Distance)	50	13	28	44	61	41	75	90	88
Near by (See Figures)	29	4	35	27	21	35	8	5	-
Elsewhere in Inner City	12	64	29						
				28	19	24	17	3	12
Further Afield (Same City)	10	18	8						
(N)	(173)	(245)	(72)	(160)	(194)	(197)	(181)	(295)	(34)

Outer City Sample (%)

	Selly Oak			Perry Barr		
	White	Asian		White	Asian	A/C
In Eastern Ward or Walking Distance	51	49	In Ward or Walking Distance	86	52	57
In Western Ward or Walking Distance	37	30	Elsewhere in Inner City	10	35	43
Elsewhere in Inner City	12	21				
Further Afield	-	-	Further Afield	5	13	-
(N)	(147)	(57)		(166)	(23)	(21)

[a] Afro-Caribbean

Table 8.4: Effects of Income, Status and Ethnic
Group Upon Consultation Patterns [a]

	Household Income	Social Class
'High' (Social Class I-III)	22%	33%
'Low' (Social Class IV, V)	38%	34%

	White	Asian	Afro-Caribbean
'Ethnic Group'	24%	36%	27%

Combined Effects	White	Asian	Afro-Caribbean
High Social Class	23	35	15
Low Social Class	26	37	33
High Income	19	29	17
Low Income	33	45	37
(N)	(356)	(370)	(128)

[a] Probability of male respondent having visited GP
    in the previous month. Income classes are
    divided at the grand median.

and Asian respondents while in Perry Barr (Figure
8.3) the differences between white and black
respondents are substantial.

By referring back to Table 8.2 to consider
another aspect of registration, it would appear that
the unequal distribution of Asian GPs has a powerful
effect on registration patterns. Many of the
doctors attended from Perry Barr in Handsworth are
of Asian origin, and of course it is a well-known
area of settlement for immigrants who may have moved
out to the relative suburbia of Perry Barr but
retained their GP links. This latter is unlikely
to be the reason for the Wolverhampton distribution
but there few of the nearest GPs were of Asian
origin, which would support the primary hypothesis.
The same explanation would fit the distribution
observed in Deritend (Figure 8.4) where virtually

Figure 8.3: Location and Usage of Doctors in North West Birmingham

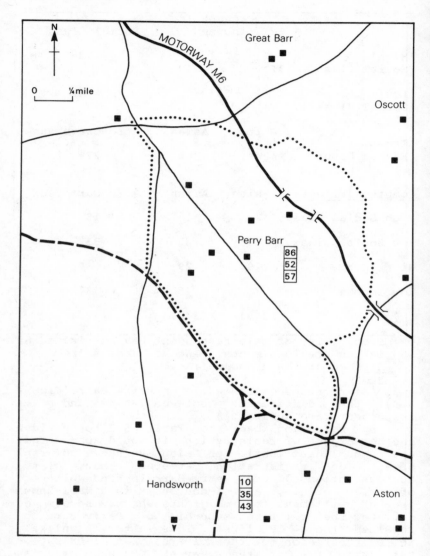

Ethnic Minorities and Primary Health Care

Figure 8.4: Location and Usage of Doctors in South Central Birmingham

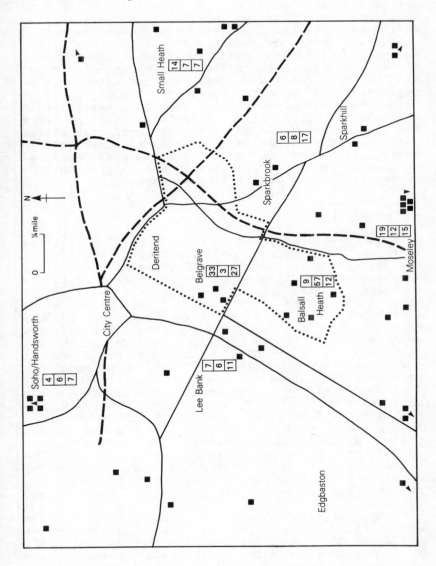

203

all the Asian registrations inside the ward are with one of the five practices in the southern area, four out of five of whom were Asian in origin compared to none of those in the north-western part. Afro-Caribbean registrations are dispersed more around classical areas of immigrant settlement, with a secondary focus in Moseley, again suggestive of either some continuity of registration or of difficulty in finding a local practice with which to register. In general, therefore, one is confident that these data demonstrate sufficient variation in distribution (even allowing for what Phillips terms the behaviour of "boundedly rational satisfiers who do not possess complete information") in registration to indicate a less than expected evenness, or more precisely, the operation of a system leading to ethnic disadvantage.

USE OF GP SERVICE

It is sometimes stated that ethnic minorities represent a 'burden' on the health services by making excessive demands. Certainly the survey demonstrated that Asian households were more likely to have visited their GP in the last year, and to have visited more frequently (Table 8.1). Afro-Caribbeans ('West Indians') were not significantly more likely to have needed a doctor although those who had done so tended to have been more frequently, often for long-standing conditions or for repeat prescriptions. However, whites were much more likely to have bypassed the GP by visiting hospital 'out patient' or 'emergency' clinics while these services were used by ethnic minorities only following referral by their G.P. Further, while Asians were most likely to have had a domiciliary visit, Afro-Caribbeans were least likely to have called the GP out, and white responses were close to those of Asians. Given the larger number of children in Asian households, one might reasonably expect them to be more likely to need a domiciliary visit.

Equally, it should be added that, at least according to respondents, few of their visits to the GP were for 'vague or poorly described symptoms'. This suggests that the visits were genuinely based on need and stemmed more from physical ailments than psychological problems. Indeed most of the psychological-based consultations were reported by white respondents. While it is accepted that there may be cultural differences in 'presenting symptoms', particularly as regards mental health, it was expected that physical presentations of mental conditions would be reported in such a form as to be considered 'vague or poorly described'.

In order to ascertain the relative significance of deprivation induced by 'race', income, and socio-economic status, these three variables were used to analyse frequency of attendance at the GP surgery. Reasons for attendance (as indicated above) do vary, most especially when gender is taken into account, depending especially on female fertility and consequently it has been chosen to illustrate this by reference only to males who overwhelmingly attended for 'short-term illness' (and for whom there were few 'ethnic' differences in reasons for attending). Table 8.4 illustrates the likelihood of having attended the GP's surgery in the (winter) months previous to the interview. While there are problems in interpreting this as being related to morbidity (that is, real illness and need), Collins and Klein [22] have shown that it is a fair proxy for relative morbidity albeit under-estimating the extent of need to a considerable extent. Their data also indicated that there were not great differences between most socio-economic groups in 'access' but they did not tackle the question of ethnicity. It therefore has to be assumed that these figures do in some sense give an estimate of health and need for primary care, as well as demonstrating usage. Certainly the directions of the (non-'racial') trends are in such a fashion as to support such an interpretation.

Table 8.4 demonstrates clearly that a division (if relatively crude) on social class lines gives little discrimination on health service usage, but that those of above average income make significantly lower use of their GP. Irrespective of income, the order of magnitude between three coarse groupings of 'social race' is similar. Evidently, income patterns and social status (for those in employment) are subject to the effects of racial discrimination in the sphere of employment, black people generally receiving less income or lower status jobs for equivalent qualifications [23]. Consequently the second part of the table, where the 'combined effects' are presented demonstrates that the few Afro-Caribbean respondents who had achieved higher income or occupational status have in fact significantly lower usage rates than white, and that social class for Asians is not necessarily cognate with income. Since Asian households are generally

larger they may contain more than one income-earner
but the higher income needs to be set against a
larger number of 'consumers', thereby aggravating
this disadvantage.

PREVENTIVE MEDICINE

The acknowledged link between 'ethnic group'
membership and rates of morbidity has caused
considerable professional concern in the field of
maternal and child health, especially as relates to
perinatal morbidity [24-27]. Much of the debate in
this field has revolved around partly formed notions
about cultural barriers to acceptance, and
differential uptake, of 'preventive' services [28].
While this may have been the impression gained by
some health care professionals it is not necessarily
borne out by the experience of reseachers [29-31]
who have found that ethnic minority parents are very
concerned to ensure their children's welfare. Such
studies have generally found that attendance at
child welfare clinics and the uptake of immunization
is at least as high among ethnic minority groups as
it is for the white population living in the same
area [32], and not infrequently higher [33]. Where
differences have been found, it is possible to
suggest that they have arisen from a poorer standard
of professional care - for example a longer delay in
'booking' Asian mothers for hospital antenatal care
despite presenting themselves to the GP at the same
stage of pregnancy as whites. While health visitors
(as a profession who have a key role in the area of
preventive child medicine), have apparently
displayed considerable interest in the problems of
practising in a multi-racial community [34], health
authorities seem to have been slow in providing
additional training. They have largely directed
their efforts into interpreter and diet provision in
hospitals and the use of translated health education
materials [35].
    The survey data from the West Midlands
illustrate the good record of ethnic minority
parents in utilising community-based preventive
services (Table 8.5). Asian and Afro-Caribbean
parents were only marginally less likely to have
attended child health ('well baby') clinics, a
result that could fall within 'sampling error'.
Given the economic reliance on mothers working in
the Afro-Caribbean community, and the expected
restrictions on Muslim women observing purdah, one

Table 8.5:   For Those with Children Under 5:   Attendance at
Child Health Care Clinic and Percentage Immunization Uptake

	White	Asian	Afro-Caribbean
Taken to clinic	93%	90%	88%
(N)	(172)	(357)	(59)

$$x^2 = 1.58 \text{ Not Significant}$$
$$df = 2$$

	White	Asian	Afro-Caribbean
Had all vaccinations[a]	43	66	53
Had some but not all	45	22	34
Not immunized	11	9	10
	100%	100%	100%
(N)	(174)	(361)	(59)

$$x^2 = 33.1 \text{ Sig } p< 0.001$$
$$df = 4$$

[a] Diphtheria, Tetanus, Whooping Cough and Polio.
'Don't knows' excluded x^2 calculations

For those whose oldest secondary school child is a girl:
Rubella immunization

	White	Asian	Afro-Caribbean
Immunized	72	69	88
Not done	21	14	7
Don't know	7	16	4
	100%	100%	100%
(N)	(90)	(152)	(67)

$$x^2 = 15.2 \text{ Sig } 0.01 <p<0.001$$
$$df = 4$$

Table 8.6: Belief That There Are Many Conditions
For Which Traditional Remedies Are Better Than
'Conventional' Medicine

	White	Asian	Afro-Caribbean
Agree	33	24	51
Don't Know	22	24	14
Disagree	45	52	34
(N)	100% (776)	100% (734)	100% (286)

x^2 = 69.8 sig p< 0.001
df = 4

might have anticipated significantly worse
attendance rates in these areas. Conversely, uptake
of child immunization among these groups was
considerably better than those of white parents in
the survey, as also reported by Baker et al [36].
Particularly few had had only some of the
recommended innoculations, while white parents had
frequently omitted whooping cough and rubella
immunization. The majority of un-vaccinated Asian
and Afro-Caribbean children were said to be as yet
too young to have completed the course; lack of
knowledge about the process was no less common among
Asians than whites and fewer mentioned 'side-
effects' or personal reasons for refusing. A small
number of respondents indicated that their children
had been given measles, smallpox or other
vaccinations but it was not possible to discern any
'ethnic' trend in this.

ALTERNATIVE MEDICINES

There are well established traditions of 'holistic
medicine' among non-European societies, and it is
sometimes assumed or believed that Asian immigrants
in particular are resistant to 'western medicine',
preferring to rely on Unani or Ayurvedic
practitioners [37,38]. This is at least, when taken
in a derogatory way, to ignore the contribution of
Islamic science to medicine, keeping alive the
legacy of Galen during the European Dark Ages.

Further, many of the fundamentals of these traditions have echoes in European health beliefs and 'folk medicine', and more attention is now being paid officially to homeopathy and such 'alternatives' in treatments. Nonetheless, it was found that there was considerably <u>less</u> support for 'traditional' and non-western methods among the Asian resondents than could perhaps have been expected.

At the level of attitudes, as opposed to reported behaviour, one found (Table 8.6) high levels of support for the statement that "there are many conditions for which traditional remedies are better", at least among Afro-Caribbean and white respondents: the majority of Asians actively disagreed. Hakims and Vaids may be active in Bradford or London although little evidence has been found for this [39], but only 2 per cent of Asian respondents in this survey had consulted one in the previous year. This might be contrasted with the 3.7% of whites who had visited an osteopath or similar alternative practitioner. Similarly some 1.8% of Asians had patronised a herbalist compared with just under 0.5% of white respondents. Perhaps most surprising was the finding that 6.5% of Afro-Caribbeans had been to a herbalist, and 17% to a private (conventional) doctor compared to only 8% of whites (7% of Asians). While this latter finding is in line with Weightman's report [40], it is remarkable that a group which is generally regarded as highly disadvantaged should feel that the NHS cannot provide adequately for its needs. Asians, on the other hand, although informally expected to be more likely to seek 'second opinions', did not prove to be so doing.

CONCLUSIONS

This study does not purport to produce a definitive statement on the use of health services by ethnic minorities. Indeed, it may be suggested that no such statement is possible. There are clearly differences between the communities in the West Midlands and those in London or the Yorkshire/ Manchester conurbation from which previous conclusions have been drawn. There are also variations between locations in the West Midlands, some arising from the 'class position' of areas and others perhaps from the nature of minority settlement (for example, Muslim or Punjabi Sikh Asians). In general, however, it is possible to demonstrate both that ethnic minorities do not make excessive or unreasonable demands upon the curative health services and that they have a positive and 'healthy' attitude towards the preventive services. Where there is higher usage it can be demonstrated to be linked to sociological or geographical inequalities such as income or environment which also affect the usage by white communities. These inequalities bear more heavily upon the black communities, because of the processes engendered by and termed as racism, and these processes of disadvantagement operate in the health service as in other spheres of life. Poor standards of professional treatment (which includes a failure to communicate or propensity to 'treat' the patient not the illness') or its perception may be allied with problems of culture which reduce the efficacy of the 'health delivery system'. It seems to be untrue that minority parents are 'pathogenic' in their approach to preventive services. Undoubtedly there are barriers or shortcomings on the patients side, but these exist universally and it is or should be the concern of the professional to understand and overcome these rather than to reject the case. Training, understanding and awareness are the key ingredients and research exists to feed these processes of development. It will do this better if it ceases to regard minorities as problems in themselves but regards them as individuals with needs in a context of structures of disadvantage.

REFERENCES

1. Johnson, M. (1984) Ethnic minorities and health: a review, Journal Royal College of Physicians, Vol. 18, pp. 228-230
2. Dodge, J.S. (1969) The Fieldworker in Immigrant Health, Staples Press.
3. Evans, D. I. and Blair, P.M., (1976) Neonatal screening in haemaglobinopathy, Archives of Disease in Childhood, Vol. 51, pp. 127
4. Goel, K. M. (1981) Reduced prevalence of rickets in Asian children in Glasgow, Lancet, Vol. 2, pp. 405
5. Qureshe, B. (1981) Transcultural medicine Pulse Magazine, October 29, November 5, November 12 (supplements)

6. Henley, A. (1979) The Asian Patient in Hospital and at Home, Pitman Medical, London
7. Wandsworth Community Relations Council (1978) Asians and the Health Service, Wandsworth Council for Community Relations, London
8. Torkington, P. (1983) The Racial Politics of Health, Merseyside Area Profile Group, Department of Sociology, Liverpool University
9. Birmingham Community Health Council (1981) 6/10 Could Do Better, Central Birmingham Community Health Council, Birmingham
10. Bolden, K. (1981) Inner Cities, Royal College of General Practitioners Occasional Paper, No. 19
11. DHSS (1980) Inequalities in Health, HMSO, London
12. Rathwell, T. (1984) General practice, ethnicity and health services delivery, Social Science and Medicine, Vol. 19, pp. 123-130
13. Clarke, M., and Clayton, D.G. (1983) Quality of obstetric care provided for Asian Immigrants in Leicestershire, British Medical Journal, Vol. 286, pp. 621
14. Rahman, S.W. (1982) An urban group practice in a mainly Asian community, Update, Vol. 24, pp. 617.
15. Ronalds, C., Vaughan, J.P., and Sprackling, P. (1977) Asian mothers use of general practitioner and maternal/child welfare services, Journal of the Royal College of General Practitioners, Vol. 27, pp. 281
16. Jarman, B. (1981) A Survey of Primary Care in London, Royal College of General Practitioners, Occasional Paper, No. 16.
17. Baker, M.R., Bandaranayake, R., and Schweiger, M.S. (1984) Differences in rate of uptake and immunisation among ethnic groups, British Medical Journal, Vol. 288, pp. 1075-1078
18. Filby, I. (1984) A Study of Interpreters in the West Midlands, West Midlands Regional Health Authority
19. Johnson, M. and Cross, M. (1984) Surveying Service Users in a Multi-racial Area, Centre for Research in Ethnic Relations, Warwick University

Ethnic Minorities and Primary Health Care

20. Blakemore, K. (1982) Health and illness among the elderly of minority ethnic groups, Health Trends, Vol. 14, pp. 69
21. Phillips, D.R. (1981) Contemporary Issues in the Geography of Health Care, Geobooks, Norwich
22. Collins, E. and Klein, R, (1980) Equity and the NHS: self-reported morbidity, access and primary care, British Medical Journal, Vol. 281, pp. 1111
23. Brown, C. (1984) Black and White Britain, Heinemann/Policy Studies Institute, London
24. Birmingham CHC (1981) op. cit.
25. Clarke, M. and Clayton, D. (1983) op. cit.
26. Save the Children Fund (1984) Asian Mother and Baby Campaign, Save the Children/Health Education Council/Department of Health and Social Security, London
27. Terry, P.B., Condie, R.G. and Settatree, R.S., (1980) Analysis of ethnic differences in perinatal statistics, British Medical Journal, Vol. 281, pp. 1307.
28. Baker, M. et al (1984) op. cit
29. Clarke, M. and Clayton, D. (1983) op. cit.
30. Currer, C. (1983) The Mental Health of Pathan Mothers in Bradford, Unpublished Report, Department of Sociology, Warwick University
31. Goodenough, S. (1984) Personal Communication
32. Ronalds, C. et al (1977) op. cit.
33. Hood, C. (1970) Children of West Indian Immigrants, Institute of Race Relations/Oxford University Press, Oxford
34. Johnson, M. (1983) Race and Health Bibliography 4, Research Unit on Ethnic Relations, Aston University, Birmingham
35. Austen, R., Cross, M., and Johnson, M. (1984) Unequal and Under Five, VOLCUF
36. Baker, M. et al (1984) op. cit.
37. Eagle, R. (1980) Your friendly neighbourhood hakim, World Medicine, Vol. 15, pp. 21
38. Aslam, M. and Healey (1983) Asiatic medicine, Update, Vol. 27, pp. 1043.
39. Currer, C. (1983) op. cit.
40. Weightman, G. (1977) Poor Man's Harley Street, New Society, 20th October, pp. 118

212

Chapter 9

DOES RACE AFFECT HOSPITAL USE?

John Griffith, Peter Wilson and Philip Tedeschi

INTRODUCTION

The relationship between race and hospital use in
the United States (US) is complicated by inter-
correlation with demographic, economic, and social
variables known to impact upon utilisation. As
these variables have changed, the relationship
between race and hospital use appears also to have
altered. Earlier evidence suggesting that whites
use hospitals more than blacks has given way to more
recent findings that reverse the relationship [1,2].
     The conventional explanation for this reversal
is that earlier barriers to access, both financial
and cultural, have given way to the combined impact
of Medicaid and Medicare, the disappearance of legal
segregation, and the attenuation of many forms of
extra-legal discrimination. As a consequence,
black use rates have risen to a level commensurate
with black need; both being considerably higher
than those found in the white populations.
     Substantial differences between white and
blacks in the US have been reported on a broad range
of health status indicators including general and
infant mortality rates, disease specific prevalence
and incidence rates, self perception of health
status, limitation of activity, source of ambulatory
care, dental visits, use of preventive health
services, and use of nursing homes [3,4]. The
direction of these differences is generally such as
to suggest greater need, both met and unmet, on the
part of the black population.

Reprinted with permission of authors and publisher
from Peter Wilson, John R. Griffith, and Philip
Tedeschi 'Does Race Affect Hospital Use?', American
Journal of Public Health, Vol. 75, 1985, pp. 263-269

Does Race Affect Hospital Use?

The research reported in this paper has the objective of identifying some of the reasons for race specific hospital use differences. Of principle concern is geographic location and its impact upon use. Blacks, however, have locational patterns substantially different from whites. For example, more than 50% of US blacks live in the South, particularly the rural South, with another large proportion living in large, non-Southern Standardized Metropolitan Statistical Areas (SMSA). Hospital use differentials are well documented at both the regional level and between urban and rural settings. In addition to these large area differences, small area studies generally demonstrate substantial use rate variation [5,6]. The failure to control for location raises the possibility that place and race are being confounded. Not only does this weaken cross-sectional comparisons but to the degree that migratory patterns are different, it confuses trend analyses.

This research focuses upon race specific hospital use in 23 Michigan communities, by distinguishing firstly between the effects of race and location upon hospital use and then proceeding to investigate use differences in terms of characteristics of the communities and their race specific populations. The findings reported suggest a number of implications for the complex relationships among use, access, and need.

DATA SOURCES

Hospitals in Michigan voluntarily submit patient discharge data to the Michigan Health Data Corporation, a consortium of 14 groups from the public and private sectors involved in health care provision, financing and policy making. These data are supplemented through co-operative arrangements with adjacent states enabling the capture of virtually all hospital use by the population of the lower peninsula of Michigan (approximately 9 million people).

The population is divided into hospital service communities, each with a set of zip (postal) codes and included population, grouped together because the hospitals in the trade centre provide the plurality of hospitalisations for patients in each of the zip codes. Zip code populations are derived from US Census figures for zip codes. Racial proportions come from US Census figures for small census areas allocated and aggregated to zip codes [7].

The 60 hospital communities or 'clusters' that result range from 20 to 750 thousand in population and involve from 1 to 18 hospitals. Each cluster is an attempt to capture a working health system in the sense that the hospital care for the population is largely (60%-90%) provided by the local institution. For this reason, the characteristics of the community can be reasonably expected to affect the levels and kinds of hospital care delivered.

Twenty-three of the 60 hospital clusters were chosen for this study. In order to be included, a cluster had to have a minimum population of 2,500 reported for races other than white, and less than 5% of its discharges of unknown race. In Michigan, over 95% of persons reporting race other than white are black. Two per cent report Hispanic origin and are included here as 'other than white'. For convenience, races other than white are referred to as 'black'.

Based on the characteristics of admission with unknown race compared to admission where race is known, the National Center for Health Services Research has concluded that 'unknowns' are probably distributed by race in the same proportions as 'knowns' [8]. This reasoning was followed here but the 5% limit was chosen to minimise the possibility that the lack of racial identification was deliberate and therefore biasing. The Institute of Medicine concluded that racial identification on medical abstracts was 94.5% reliable, with most of the problem being the omission of racial identifiers in the underlying medical record [9]. Based on these findings, the authors are satisfied that these discharge data are sound. The choice of 1980 as the period of analysis enabled the use of US Census counts and to derive high quality estimates of race specific small area populations.

The 23 clusters have a combined population of 5,753,000, of which 4,548,000 or 79% are white, and 1,205,000 or 21% are black. As might be expected, Detroit and many of its suburbs are included. The seven-county Southeast Michigan area has 13 communities in it, 22% of the total 60 clusters. Nine of these, or 39% are also in the black set of 23. Over 96% of the total black population of Michigan resides in our 23 clusters.

Does Race Affect Hospital Use?

METHODOLOGY

The analyses are conducted upon the non-obstetric patient day rates, discharge rates, and lengths of stay for the 23 clusters, standardised for the age structure of the total Michigan population using six age categories (0-14, 15-29, 30-44, 45-64, 65-74, 75 and over).

The first step was to examine the patient day rates of whites and blacks by pooling the 23 clusters, and comparing their individual values. The impact of location on the two racial groups by correlation was tested by examining four components — the total patient day rate, discharges and length of stay for surgical and nonsurgical cases.

The next stage examined the individual community differences through multi-variate analysis using two linear models. In 'Model One' the question of access is examined indirectly, through cluster measures of supply variables.

Model One has five independent variables: the population of the community, the percentage of the population that is black, the acute bed to population ratio, the surgeon to population ratio, and the non-surgeon physician to population ratio. For the three supply variables, cross community traffic was accommodated by attributing distant physicians and beds to local populations based on the proportion of local use of distant resources. For example, if the population of Community A represented 7% of the bed days in the hospitals in Community B, 7% of Community B beds are attributed to Community A. Similar allocations are made for physicians, with surgeons distributed on the basis of surgical admissions, and non-surgeon physicians on the basis of medical patient days (See Appendix A). Population size and per cent black were included to detect any systematic differences between urban and rural environments or effects which depend upon the impact of the black population, for example, the emergence of a distinct medical care sub-system. Table 9.1 displays the range of values for these variables in the communities.

It is generally accepted that supply variables are positively associated with hospital use. In Michigan, rural use tends to be higher than urban. The impact of 'per cent black' is unknown, but it may be that higher black densities lead to special

Does Race Affect Hospital Use?

access situations such as higher numbers of black
doctors, the existence of black hospitals, or
'ghettos' of under-served populations.

Although Model One variables are estimated for
the whole community, it is possible that a
differential impact exists between races. Black
use may increase more rapidly than white use as
these resources become more available. It was
hypothesised that the Model One variables would show
the same regression relationships for blacks and
whites.

In Model Two, the impact of four population
characteristics on use was examined. These four
measures, discussed below, are available on a race
specific basis.

Morbidity
Measures of health status for small area populations
are difficult to construct both conceptually and
operationally. Use has been made of the
standardised mortality ratio (SMR), and index of
actual to expected mortality, controlling for age
and sex. Race specific ratios were prepared by
county by the Michigan Department of Public Health,
and were translated to communities based upon
county-community population coincidence.

Education
The percentage of the population over age 25 which
has not graduated from high school is used to
measure educational attainment. This variable, and
the two that follow, are from US Census File STF3B,
information from the 20% long form sample,
aggregated to zip codes. Furthermore the
information was aggregated to the level of the
communities, themselves sets of zip codes.

Unemployment
Unemployment is measured as the percentage of the
adult population seeking but unable to find work.
In 1980, the latest recession was well underway in
Michigan, but many unemployed were still covered
under employment related health insurance.

Poverty
Poverty is measured as the percentage of
families below the 1979 Federal poverty level

standard, but many unemployed were still covered under employment related insurance.

As Table 9.1 indicates, the ranges are striking both within and between the race specific populations. On average, blacks have a death rate 6% higher than white, 12% fewer of adults have graduated from high school, about twice the proportion of the population is unemployed, and almost three times the proportion of families is below the poverty level. However, as the correlation co-efficients indicate, while white and black populations have extraordinarily different socio-economic characteristics, the relative community standing for the race specific populations are highly correlated.

The zero order relations between the race specific education, unemployment, and poverty variables indicated substantial multi-collinearity among these measures of socio-economic status:

```
White
High School (WHS)     1.00           Rho (.05) = .42
Unemployed (WUn)      -.65  1.00
Poverty (WPov)        -.54   .40  1.00
Non-white              .67  -.31  -.56   1.00
High School (NWHS)    -.67   .59   .37   -.65   1.00
Unemployed (NWUn)     -.46   .30   .73   -.78    .64   1.00
Poverty (NWPov)       WHS   WUn  WPov   NWHS   NWUn  NWPov
```

A principal components analysis using the least squares method was performed to produce the factor socio-economic status (SES). Factor loadings were uniformly high and the variance explained was 79%. Table 9.1 includes a description of the factors.

The hypothesis is that these factors will have similar co-efficients for each race, and it is hypothesised that justifying for these values will substantially reduce inter-racial differences.

FINDINGS

Table 9.2 shows the 1980 non-obstetric patient day rates for each race in the 23 communities. In only 5 places is black use lower than white. The median difference is more than 200 days per 1,000 population additional care to blacks. In aggregate (Table 9.3) the 23 communities have a white non-obstetrical use rate of 1,061 patient days per thousand population and a black rate of 1,651, both

Does Race Affect Hospital Use?

Table 9.1: Community Characteristics

Characteristic	Minimum	Maximum	Mean	Std. Dev.	White/Non-white Correlation[a] (Spearman's Rho)
Population	20,303	860,630	249,550	219,110	
% Non-white	2	72	13	15	
Acute beds/1000	3.3	6.0	4.5	0.8	
Surgeons/1000	.24	.56	.35	.08	
Non-surgeons/1000	.41	.96	.65	.16	
Morbidity (standardised mortality ratio)					
White	.81	1.07	.97	.07	.57
Non-White	.29	1.36	1.03	.30	.67
Education (% non-high school graduates)					
White	21	55	32		.59
Non-white	26	62	44		.73
Unemployment (% of labour force)					
White	5.4	15.2	10.0	2.4	.69
Non-white	10.5	28.5	19.0	5.2	
Poverty (% families below 1979 US standard)					
White	4.4	19.4	8.8	3.7	
Non-white	11.6	36.5	22.1	7.0	
SES (Factor)[b]					
White	-2.2	4.0	2.0	1.3	
Non-white	-6.2	2.1	-2.1	2.2	

[a] p (.01) = .54
[b] A factor for education, unemployment, and poverty. See text. Weights were: Unemployment, .86; poverty, .90; Education, .90. Eigen value =2.37 Variance explained 78.9%.

Table 9.2: Individual Values of Age Adjusted
Non-obstetric Patient Day Rates 23 Michigan
Communities

White	Blacks	Difference
855.7	621.1	-234.69
999.9	791.5	-208.42
1160.2	954.8	-205.43
1213.7	1045.5	-168.18
992.0	935.3	-56.76
969.5	986.2	16.72
838.4	896.2	57.83
904.9	996.2	91.28
1722.9	1840.9	117.97
1021.2	1148.4	127.26
1078.8	1262.6	183.74
1292.0	1518.8	226.81
1203.8	1437.8	234.02
834.1	1144.2	310.08
1169.2	1482.7	313.58
791.9	1171.0	379.17
1057.3	1470.1	412.78
832.3	1267.2	434.93
1238.5	1691.1	452.61
1018.3	1507.2	488.92
1324.7	1826.1	501.40
1104.6	1684.0	579.39
1325.6	2739.0	1413.40

age adjusted to the state population. Differences
for discharge rates are relatively similar; those
for length of stay relatively smaller.

Earlier studies on the Michigan data base had
established the profound influence of location upon
levels of hospital use. Non-obstetrical patient
day rates vary across communities with a range
exceeding two to one. Communities that are high
(or low) on one dimension of hospital use tend to
maintain that standing on other dimensions of use.
High Blue Cross use accompanies high Medicaid use,
aged with young, surgery with medicine, admission
rates with length of stay [10,11]. Based on these
findings, it was expected that race specific
hospital use differences would narrow when
individual communities, rather than aggregate, were
compared.

Does Race Affect Hospital Use?

This expectation was confirmed as illustrated in Table 9.3. The top part of the Table presents race specific use for the study populations treated as aggregate. By ignoring community of residence one has what is in effect a statewide rate. The bottom part of the Table shows the individual values and the mean rates for the 23 community populations. The pooled age adjusted patient day rate difference is 56%; the individual community mean difference is 22%. Similar reductions in difference are seen for both discharge rate and length of stay.

Some of the difference is attributable to a single cluster, where black use is over twice white use (2,739 patient days, 268 discharges per 1,000 population). If that cluster is removed, the black means are 1,259 patient days/1,000 population and 152 discharges/1,000 population, 17% and 15% above the similarly adjusted white rates. The black standard deviations are significant. The questionable cluster is more than four standard deviations from the mean patient day rate and 2.8 standard deviations from the mean discharge rate. The community is one of Michigan's poorer, but it is not an outlier on the dependent variables considered below. No evidence is available on the cause of the high values for this community.

The reason why the race difference is reduced is that in Michigan, as in the US, blacks are not uniformly distributed among communities. A higher proportion of blacks live in communities with high levels of hospitalisation. However, these high levels of hospitalisation are experienced by both the white and black populations of the communities.

Table 9.4 indicates the correlations between white and non-black use for the total non-obstetrical patient day rate and its components analysed into medical and surgical services by discharge rate and length of stay. Seven of the nine cells show correlation well beyond the 95% confidence level. Clearly, whatever drives hospital use at the community level acts upon both racial groups.

However, race specific patient day rates track at different levels, with black use higher than white use. Figure 9.1 illustrates the relationship between the white and black patient day rates across the 23 communities. The black rate ranges from 73%

Does Race Affect Hospital Use?

Figure 9.1: Black Day Rate as Percentage of White
Rate, 23 Communities

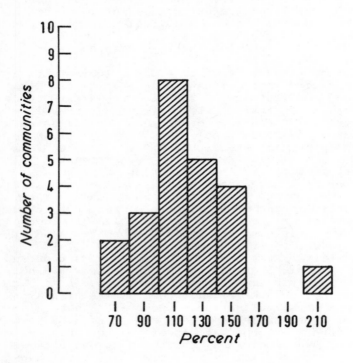

able 9.3   The Effect of Location on Race Specific
ospital Use Differences: 23 Michigan Communities

| | 23 Communities Aggregated (a) | | | |
	White	Non-white	Difference	$\frac{\text{non-white}}{\text{white}}$ x 100
atient days er 1000 opulation age adjusted)	1061	1651	156%	
ischarges per 000 population age adjusted)	129	174	135%	
bserved length f stay	8.3	9.2	110%	

a)   Sum of all patient days/sum of all population,
ge adjusted

| | 23 Communities: Mean Rates (b) | | | |
	White	Non-white	Difference	$\frac{\text{non-white}}{\text{white}}$ x 100
atient days er 1000 opulation age adjusted)	1085[c] (216.3)	1323 (455.2)	122%	
ischarges er 1000 opulation age adjusted)	139 (20.4)	157 (46.9)	113%	
bserved length f stay	7.9 (1.11)	8.1 (1.12)	103%	

b) Sum of individual community rates/23
    Standard deviations in parentheses

c] Difference in means significant
    with P<.05, Student's t-test

Does Race Affect Hospital Use?

Table 9.4:   White and Black Hospital Use
Correlations: 23 Communities Spearman's Rho

	Patient day rate	Discharge rate	Average length of Stay
Total non-obstetrical	.68**	.57**	.73**
Surgical	.77**	.60**	.40
Medical	.51*	.44*	.87**

P(.05) = .42(*)
P(.01) = .55(**)

to 207% of the white rate. This raises the question
of why the community by community relationship
between the rates swings through a range approaching
3 to 1.
     The patient day rate of a population is the
product of its admission rate and average length of
stay. As Table 9.3 indicates, race specific length
of stay differences, important at the national level
and for our 23 communites when aggregated,
essentially evaporate once location is controlled.
More detailed analysis, not shown here, indicates
that whites and blacks have about the same case mix,
at least as it impacts length of stay, and are kept
in the hospital about the same length of time.
While hospital stays are similar, the arrival rate
at the hospital differs markedly.
     Figure 9.2 displays age and service specific
discharge rates for the white and black populations
of the 23 communities. Table 9.5 shows means and
tests of significance. The first interesting
finding is that the white and black populations,
when age adjusted, are at the same risk for surgical
admissions, but the black population is much more
likely to be hospitalised for medical (non-surgical)
reasons. Most of the difference in patient day
rates can be attributed to the difference in medical
discharge rates. This finding conflicts with other
reports that blacks receive less surgery than
whites [12]. The age sensitivity of the comparison
may be a cause of the differing conclusions.
     The second interesting finding is that for both
medicine and surgery, there is a strong age specific
flavour to hospital use differences. Black medical
discharge rates are higher in every age cohort.

Does Race Affect Hospital Use?

Figure 9.2: Age-specific White and Black Discharge
Rates 23 Michigan Communities

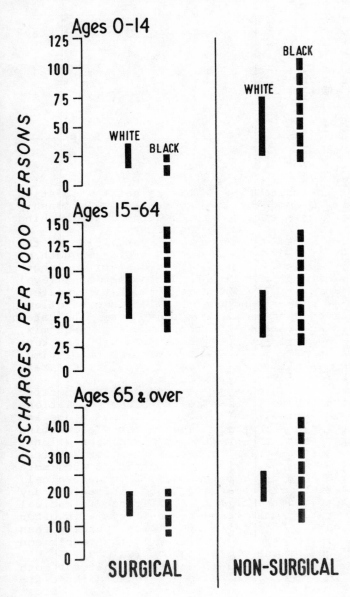

Table 9.5: Age, Race and Service Specific Discharge Rates: Means for 23 Communities

Discharges per 1000 population	0-14			15-64			64+			age adjusted total		
	white	black	% diff.	white	black	% diff.	white	black	% diff.	white	black	% diff.
Medical	48	54	113%	53[a]	74	140	207[a]	236	144	66[a]	84	127
	(12.2)	(21.4)		(11.2)	(28.7)		(22.8)	(63.6)		(11.39)	(27.07)	
Surgical	26[a]	16	62%	77	83	108	163[a]	144	88	73	73	100
	(6.00)	(4.96)		(12.4)	(29.6)		(17.4)	(31.4)		(10.52)	(22.03)	

[a] Difference in means significant with P < .05, Student's t-test

Does Race Affect Hospital Use?

Table 9.6: Values for Regressions of Race Specific
Age Adjusted Non-obstetric Patient Day Rates Against
Access and Supply Factors - 23 Michigan Communities

Indep. Variable	White Coeff.	t Stat	Black Coeff.	t Stat
Constant	158.2	.54	-53	.06
Size				
Population	.0003	1.05	.0007	.89
Pct.				
Non-white	1.17	0.28	-1.35	-.12
Acute Beds	158.11	2.63	163.3	1.27
Surgeons	-86.4	-.18	-482.3	-.37
Non-Surgeons	230.8	.87	681.7	.95
F		5.0		1.66
R^2		.60		.32

They are 40% higher for black adults aged 15 to 64.
Approximately two-thirds of the population is in
this age group. Conversely, surgical discharge
rates differ by age group, they have less in the
childhood and aged years. When the data are
adjusted to the Michigan population the difference
in surgery disappears. The most striking
difference is among children. Black children use
only two-thirds the surgery of whites. It is hard
to believe that their needs are proportionately
met.

ANALYSIS

The analysis deals with two questions raised by the
findings:
1.   Whether general community characteristics -
     size, per cent black, and health care resources
     - act uniformly on black and white use.
2.   Whether individual characteristics - mortality
     and economic status - act uniformly on black
     and white use.
These questions were approached in terms of two
multi-variate regression models, the first
incorporating community and supply variables and the
second socio-economic and health status variables
which have been hypothesised to affect demand.

Does Race Affect Hosptial Use?

Table 9.7: Values for Regression of Race Specific Age Adjusted Non-obstetric Patient Day Rates Against Mortality and Socio-economic Factors - 23 Michigan Communities (t Statistics in Parentheses)

| | Patient Day Rate (per 1000 pop., age adjusted, non-obstetrical) | | | |
Dependent Variable	White	Black	White and Black	White and Black
Independent Variable	(n-23)	(n=23)	(n=46)	(n=46)
Constant	−397	321	181	120
	(1.8)	(1.1)	(.9)	(.6)
Dummy (NW=1)				118
				(.9)
SMR	1662	988	1022	1026
	(3.5)	(3.8)	(5.2)	(5.2)
SES	−62.9	7.5	−29.7	−13.3
	(2.4)	(.2)	(1.9)	(.6)
F	16.0	7.1	18.3	12.5
R^2	.62	.42	.46	.47

P < .05 fpr F > 2.0

Does Race Affect Hospital Use?

Table 9.8: Values for regression of Race
Specific Non-obstetric Age Adjusted Patient Day
Rates Against Mortality and Individual Socio-economic
Variables - 23 Michigan Communities

Dependent Variable	White Coef.	t Stat	Black Coef.	Non-white t Stat
Constant	587	.64	1298	1.32
SMR	1314.6	1.66	1086	4.10
High School %	-12.6	-1.69	-13.3	-.29
Unemplo %	13.5	.46	30.6	1.53
Poverty %	-5.9	- .44	-42.0	-2.26
F	8.1		5.6	
R^2	.64		.55	

Model One
Regression results for white and black age adjusted
non-obstetrical patient day rates against supply
factors are shown in Table 9.6. Regressions were
also run on the community ratio of black to white
use (not shown). Of the three regressions, only that
for the white patient day rate was significant and
that was because of the strong relationship between
use and acute bed supply. The bed supply had the
highest statistic in the other two as well (1.3. or
p approximately .8). Multiple R^2 values of .32
and .29 for the black and ratio variables fell well
short of significance for 17 degrees of freedom.
    Variation in supply of resource, either beds or
physicians, has no significant power to explain the
variation in black use, even though beds are
significant in explaining white use. Size of the
total community and per cent black have no
significance in explaining either white or black
use.

Model Two
Table 9.7 displays the co-efficients for regressions
of the race specific rates for four different
formulations. The first two are the race specific
age adjusted, non-obstetrical patient day rates.
The third and fourth are the race specific rates
combined into a single set of 46, and run with and
without a dummy variable for race. Each regression
uses standardised mortality and the SES factor as
independent variables. All regressions were

229

significant. The white rate was somewhat better explained than the black rate, because of a significant negative association with SES.

In all the regressions, increased mortality is significantly associated with greater hospital use. At the means, a 10% increase in white mortality is associated with a 15% increase in the white patient day rate. A 10% increase in black mortality is associated with an 8% increase in the black rate.

SES factor differences affect white use rates significantly but do not influence black use. As white SES improves, the patient day rate is depressed. At the means, a 10% increase in white SES lowers the white patient day rate by 1%. When the components of the SES factor were used individually, both SMR and poverty emerged as significant for black patient day rates (Table 9.8). For the white population, no single factor was significant although overall R^2 = .64 and p<.01.

Regressions were run on all 46 patient day rates with and without a dummy variable for race. The dummy variable itself is not significant and its inclusion does not substantially affect the co-efficients on SMR and SES. The null hypothesis, that white and black populations do not differ in their use of hospitals when SMR and SES are controlled, cannot be rejected.

Given the problematic issue of the outlier community, the regressions in Table 9.7 were run again, without substantial alteration of the results (see Appendix B).

CONCLUSIONS

The analysis began with the finding that blacks use hospitals at a rate approximately 50% higher than whites when Michigan communities with significant black populations were examined. It is not, however, the case that this 50% difference is found on a community by community basis. Although a wide range of differences was found within communities, on average the black population of a community used 22% more hospital care than the white population of the same community. The difference shrank because blacks are disproportionately represented in high use communities - communities that deliver a lot of hospital care to their population regardless of colour. The rank correlation of the white and black patient day rates was .64, well over the .01 significance level for 23 cases.

Does Race Affect Hospital use?

This left two questions. First, how black use is influenced by general community characteristics, and second, how it is influenced by individual characteristics.

It was not possible to relate either the absolute or relative levels of black use to community size, percentage of blacks in the population, or the supply of physicians or beds, although white use is associated with the bed supply. In general terms, Michigan is a state whose communities are well endowed with medical care resources and whose hospital care is well financed through a combination of public and private means. There is no evidence that under these circumstances race specific use varies systematically with supply.

A more fruitful source of explanation lay with population characteristics indicative of health and socio-economic status. The white and black populations differed dramatically across communities for each race. On average blacks were substantially lower in health and socio-economic terms than whites although there was a strong tendency for the white and black populations to be similarly ranked within the commmunity they share.

For both whites and blacks, increased standardised mortality ratio as a proxy for morbidity results in increased hospital use. Improved SES in the white population, but not the black population, decreases use. These findings suggest that hospital use differences are to some extent need driven or at least that increased need is reflected in increased use. Individual characteristics differently distributed between the races, result in different use. However, the exact impact still differs between races.

Can it be stated that hospital use remains affected by race, given the isolation of morbidity and SES differences? In terms of the statistical analysis, the answer is no. The proportion of hospital use differences in those populations leaves a non-significant residual. In other words, white and black Michigan populations with the same morbidity and SES scores do not differ significantly in their use of hospitals.

Finally, there remains the question of the degree to which observations based upon 23 Michigan communities can Be generalised to the nation. In Michigan, aggregating all black use and all white use ignores the differing population distributions and approximately doubles the difference between the races. This is because blacks are disproportionately located in high use places, and location affects hospital use. It is believed that similar errors may occur when other aggregates are compared.

The communities run the gamut from small rural to very large urban and include the variety of economic, social, and political circumstances typical of the environments shared by white and black Americans. The data base is of a very high quality not likely to be matched in many locales where significant numbers of blacks are found. Considering all the evidence, it is probably fair to say that substantial progress has been made in attenuating the significance of race as a variable directly explanatory of hospital use [13]. Indirectly, through education, poverty, and behaviour towards subgroups such as children needing surgery, racial differences clearly remain.

Further work in other geographic areas would be useful. Within this data set, exploration of the most striking remaining area of reduced black use, surgery in children, is very much in order.

APPENDIX A

One could question the allocation procedure used for the supply measures on the grounds that this approach confuses supply with demand and therefore should be avoided. The communities represent a mixed picture. The seven in southeast Michigan, near Detroit, are geographically close, but the other 16 tend to be scattered. The non-Detroit communities are generally larger cities with referral capabilities, and three or four might be considered 'tertiary'. As a result they all have net inflows of patients, and some have substantial net inflows. Other than to the 'tertiary' centres, they do not refer extensively between each other. the inflows are principally from the 23 other non-Detroit communities. Therefore, an unadjusted supply would overstate reality, and for the tertiary centres be a substantial exaggeration. The Detroit communities include three at or near tertiary levels, and are largely adjacent. A complex pattern of inter-referral exists which the authors believe on balance is better represented by adjustment than not.

Does Race Affect Hospital use?

The adjustment used in a first order approximation is the true access for any citizen, because the citizen can (and does) go outside his/her own community for care. However the full solution to this problem is formidable:

Let i = community of patient residence
         j = community of supply location
     U_{ij} = use (e.g. discharges)
     S_{ij} = supply factor (e.g. beds, doctors)
     $S_{.j}$ = total supply at location j
     a_{ij} = weight for access of i residents to
          j location
Then $S_{ij} = a_{ij} S_{.j}$

then if one assumes a_{ij} is related to actual use preference:
$$E_U = E_j a_{ij} s_j$$

$$j \ ij \ j^{a_{ij}S}.j$$

constitutes one of a set of 69 equations (one for each i) whose simultaneous solution by regression would estimate then 3,600 a_{ij}. The resulting weights can be used to calculate an effective supply,

$$S_i = {}^E a_{ij} S_{.j}{}_j$$

so far as the authors know, no one has ever carried this approach to completion. Certainly we will not, with 60 data points. This actual solution assumes that:

$$a_{ij} = U_{ij} U_{.j}$$

The authors believe this is a reasonable approximation. Over 60% of the hospital use occurs in the community of residence. The second most used community rarely captures 10%. The notion that a more refined measure would change the significance of the result seems improbable.

APPENDIX B

The regressions shown in Table 6 were also run excluding the outlier case. The results are as follows:

Constant	306.6 (.59)	445 (2.2)	328 (1.96)
Dummy	–	–	38.7 (.39)
SMR	1,568 (3.1)	788 (4.1)	825 (5.3)
SES	-65.0 (-2.4)	-5.57 (-.22)	-24.3 (1.33)
F	14.1	8.9	13.7
R^2	.60	.48	.51
Significance	<.01	<.01	<.01

REFERENCES

1. Anderson, R. and Newman, J.F. (1973) Societal and individual determinants of medical care utilization in the United States, Milband Memorial Fund Quarterly/Health and Society, Vol. 51, pp. 95-124
2. Feldstein, P.J. and German, J.J. (1975) Predicting hospital utilisation: an evaluation of three approaches, Inquiry, Vol. 2, pp. 13-36
3. US Department of Health, Education and Welfare (1979) Health United States, DHEW Publication No. (PHS) 80-1232, Washington, DC, pp. 3-29
4. Institute of Medicine (1981) Health Care in a Context of Civil Rights, National Academy Press, Washington DC
5. Wennebergm, J.E. and Gittlesohn, A. (1973) Small area variations in health care delivery, Science, Vol. 183, pp. 135-160
6. Griffith, J. (1981) Measuring community hospital services in Michigan, Health Services Research, Vol. 16, pp. 135-160
7. Thomas, W., Griffith, J. and Durance, P. (1979) The Specification of Hospital Service Communities in a Large Metropolitan Area, Technical Paper No. 5, Program and Bureau of Hospital Administration, University of Michigan, Ann Arbor

8. Department of Health and Human Services (1982) _Utilization of Short Stay Hospitals: Annual Summary for the United States_, DHSS Publication No. (PHS) 82-1725, Series 13, No. 64, Washington DC

9. National Academy of Sciences (1980) _Reliability of National Hospital Discharge Survey Data_, National Academy Press, Washington DC

10. Wilson, P. and Tedeschi, P.J. (1984) Community correlates of hospital use, _Health Services Research_, Vol. 19, pp. 333-335

11. Wilson, A. (1981) Hospital use by the ageing population, _Inquiry_, Vol. 18, pp. 332-334

12. Institute of Medicine, op. cit., pp. 50-51

13. Cordle, F. and Tyroler, H. (1974) The use of hospital medical records for epidemiological research, _Medical Care_, Vol. 12, pp. 596-610

Chapter 10

NUTRITIONAL STATUS OF BLACK COMMUNITIES IN THE
EASTERN CAPE: SOUTH AFRICA - ASSESSMENT AND
POLICY RECOMMENDATIONS

Rob Fincham

.

INTRODUCTION

The purpose of this chapter is to highlight
variations in nutrition between young black children
in metropolitan, rural and squatter communities in
the Eastern Cape, South Africa and to assess
nutrition intervention strategies appropriate to
each community. Accordingly, aspects of a
continuing nutritional surveillance programme
initiated in January 1980 are discussed along with
the policy implications of the work. The chapter
consists of three interrelated sections. The first
briefly outlines the surveillance programme while
the second provides a description of the study area.
The final section discusses the results of the
programme to date and strategies for improving
nutritional conditions where those are found to be
unsatisfactory.

THE NUTRITION SURVEILLANCE PROGRAMME

The surveillance programme has been conducted by the
Institute for Social and Economic Research (ISER) at
Rhodes University, Grahamstown, with the author as
project director. The programme arose from a
request by the Department of Health (DOH) to
ascertain conditions in the black Group Areas of
Grahamstown and among black labourers on the
surrounding white-owned commercial farms of the
Albany magisterial district (Figure 10.1).
National and international media reports of poor
nutrition and high infant mortality among young
black children suggested a totally unsatisfactory
situation. It was claimed in the media that
information from the Medical Officer of Health's
(MOH) annual report showed that one out of every
four black babies born in Grahamstown died before

Figure 10.1: The Study Area

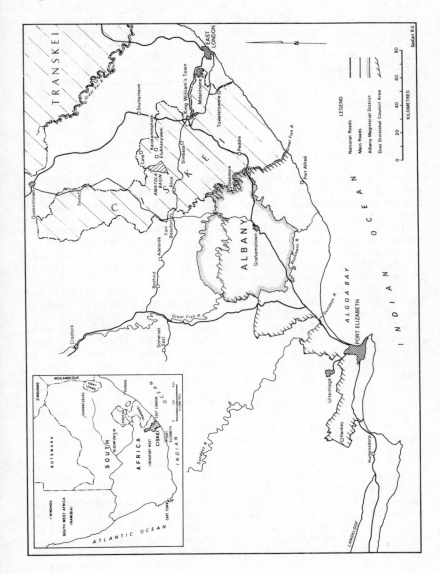

the age of twelve months. More than half the deaths of black babies were attributed directly or indirectly to malnutrition [1]. The DOH on the other hand pointed out that the MOH's statistics were misleading. The suggested infant mortality rate (IMR) of 250/1,000 live births was based on the 396 <u>registered</u> black births in Grahamstown. Since the official black population was 40,000 and the estimated black birth rate 40 per 1,000, the number of births must have been closer to 1,600 giving an IMR of 63 per 1,000 or one quarter of the IMR quoted in the news media. The DOH maintained that there was insufficient information available for an accurate assessment of nutritional conditions and IMR's since no community based studies of these factors had been undertaken.

A pilot survey of school entrants in both the urban and rural black schools of the Grahamstown area was undertaken in January 1980. It was envisaged that a nutritional survey of school entrants, a captive survey population, would also be indicative of conditions among pre-school children, a nutritionally high risk group as much previous research has indicated [2-4].

The basis of the pilot survey was a set of age dependent Boston or Harvard anthropometric measurements used to determine linear growth of children. The survey, using qualified nursing sisters from the DOH for the survey teams covered just over 3,000 children, roughly 98 per cent of school children between the ages of 5 and 9 years. The results suggested that in Grahamstown up to 60 per cent of children were at nutritional risk, that is, below the third percentile of weight and height for age. Black children of labourers on white-owned commercial farms appeared to be relatively better off with approximately one-third of children at risk.

The pilot survey showed that as many as two-thirds of children already at school were suffering from stunted growth or nutritional dwarfism. They were the children who had survived the diseases of infancy and had adapted to an environment of food scarcity. What the pilot survey did not do was to provide information on the household socio-economic conditions from which the children came or an estimate of the IMR, an important indicator of health conditions. Since the DOH felt that the survey results suggested a situation which needed attention and the ISER intended to expand its programme of nutritional surveillance, it was decided to continue with a more detailed survey programme in the Eastern Cape. The programme would however shift the focus of attention to the household level so that information about the child and its environment could be obtained as well as an idea of the IMR. The survey at the household level also provided the opportunity to measure the nutrition of children 0 to 5 years of age, the group at high risk to malnutrition and the diseases to which malnourished children succumb to more readily.

The study area is outlined in the following section with the balance of the paper devoted to a consideration of three community surveys conducted at the household level. These surveys reflect a concern with nutrition and the associated socio-economic conditions prevailing at the household level, as well as with measures to improve unsatisfactory nutritional situations.

THE STUDY AREA

The communities considered here are those of black residents in metropolitan Port Elizabeth and two Ciskeian communities, one a rural, supposedly agriculturally based community, the other a squatter community.

New Brighton and 'Little Soweto by-the-Sea' are black residential areas in metropolitan Port Elizabeth. Port Elizabeth (Figure 10.1) is the hub of industrial activity in the Eastern Cape, a depressed socio-economic region within the South African space economy [5,6]. New Brighton is fairly typical of planned black residential accommodation in the apartheid city and has a population of about 60,000 inhabitants. The basic infrastructural elements such as schools, clinics, roads, electricity and piped water are to be found in the township. Little Soweto is a spontaneous squatter settlement which has sprung up since about 1979 in response to the housing needs of migrants to the city from rural and homeland environments in the Eastern Cape. The population of approximately 80,000 live in often barely adequate housing in an environment with little infrastructural development when compared with New Brighton.

The Amatola Basin shown in Figure 10.1 consists of some 13 villages with a total population of 3,830. The Amatola is to be found in the now 'independent' Ciskei, an entity arrived at through the grand design of the apartheid policy of the present government. The historical and geographical position of Ciskei is such that for the purposes of this paper it is considered an integral part of the Eastern Cape. The Amatola community is indicative of living conditions in rural Ciskei [7,8] not beset by the immigration of people from 'white' South Africa as part of government resettlement plans in the country [9].

Tsweletewele, a squatter community approximately 25 kilometres from the port of East London is the other community studied (Figure 10.1). It has a residential population of about 5,300. An additional 1,500 are weekly commuters, work in Mdantsane and East London, and are the main source of income for the settlement [10]. The settlement is seen as temporary in the eyes of the Ciskeian authorities and little effort has been made to provide adequate basic health, sanitation and other necessary facilities.

RESULTS OF THE SURVEILLANCE PROGRAMME

Malnutrition and its Measurement

Malnutrition occurs in most of the underdeveloped world through a deficiency of essential nutrients. Such nutrients are required for the maintenance of existing tissue, the growth and regeneration of new cells and metabolic support for the range of activities in which the individual participates. If nutrients are not in sufficient supply normal physiological function becomes impossible [11]. Deficiencies can be a result of traditional dietary practices, for example vitamin deficiencies leading to Pelagra in corn-eating societies and Beri-beri in rice-eating societies. A more important general deficiency syndrome however is that of protein energy malnutrition (PEM) which in its most severe form results in Kwashiorkor and Marasmus. PEM is most common in childhood and may be responsible for the majority of paediatric hospital admissions in underdeveloped countries; it is also a major contributor to high rates of infant mortality, whether directly or indirectly in association with concurrent infection [12].

Severe malnutrition represents only part of the nutritional problems of poor communities, the so-called tip of the nutritional iceberg problem [13]. Johnston states the problem succinctly:

> Severe malnutrition requiring hospitalization and rehabilitation is appallingly striking. However it accounts for but a small proportion of infants and children who are diagnosed as malnourished. Children with chronic mild-to-moderate malnutrition suffer as well, and the long-term effects on their health and mental function may be more significant for society than the increased mortality due to severe malnutrition [14].

The critical cut off point to designate who is at risk from malnutrition is made for the purposes of this paper according to a set of international anthropometric norms called the National Centre for Health Statistics (NCHS) Percentiles [15], in essence identical in function to the Harvard norms but of more recent origin. Children falling below the third percentile of both weight-for-age (the measure used to indicate the present nutritional status of the subject, or wasting, where those below the third percentile have less than 80 per cent of expected weight for age) and height-for-age (the measure of long term nutritional status, or stunting, where the subject has less than 90 per cent of expected height for age) are regarded as being at nutritional risk. In South Africa, Hansen [16] has shown that those subjects falling below the third percentile also have clinically verifiable nutritional disorders such as inappropriate serum albumin levels, while Thomas [17] has shown that children in Ciskei not treated for malnutrition and falling below the third percentile have dramatically higher rates of mortality and morbidity than children above the third percentile.

Nutritional assessment

Tables 10.1 and 10.2 give the present and long-term nutritional status of children in the surveyed communities.

Nutritional Status of Black Communities

Table 10.1: Assessment of Weight for Age,
Children 0-5 years, all Communities, NCHS Norms

Number and Percentage below the third percentile

Locality	No. of Cases	No. < 3p	% < 3p
New Brighton	205	13	6.3
Soweto	244	20	8.2
Amatola Basin	223	29	13.0
Tsweletswele	163	70[a]	42.9

[a] These are approximate values since is was not
     always possible to verify the exact age of the
     children in Tsweletswele.

Table 10.2: Assessment of Height for Age,
Children 0-5 years, all Communities, NCHS Norms

Number and Percentage below the third percentile

Locality	No. of cases[a]	No. <3P	% <3P
New Brighton	203	34	16.7
Soweto	244	117	48.1
Amatola Basin	218	97	44.5
Tsweletswele	158	80	50.6

[a] Slight variation in the number of cases in
     Tables 10.1 and 10.2 reflect questionnaire
     response differences.

     Brown and Brown [18] suggest that if more than
15 per cent of a community's children are at risk
(that is, fall below the third percentile) then the
community has a problem and definitive steps need to
be taken to ameliorate conditions.   The weight-for-
age measures show that only Tsweletswele has greater
than 15 per cent at risk. It was also the only
community in which Frank Kwashiorkor surfaced: one
out of every ten children surveyed had verifiable
signs of the disease.   The assessment of long-term
nutrition as show in Table 10.2 revealed a marked

difference between conditions in New Brighton and the other communities. While New Brighton has approximately 15 per cent of children stunted the figure is much closer to half for all other communities.

The results suggest definite variations in nutrition. The Ciskeian communities and Little Soweto appear the worse off. While conditions in Amatola at the time of the survey appeared satisfactory, the long-term trend is one of malnourishment reflecting food scarcity. Whereas 13 per cent of the children are at risk to wasting, approximately one-third of children under the age of two are stunted and the figure rises to nearly 60 per cent of children aged 3 to 5 years.

Tsweletswele provides a depressing commentary on conditions in squatter settlements in Ciskei. It is an extremely poor environment mirrored in both the present and long-term nutritional condition of the children. Soweto seems to be little better than the Ciskeian communities in terms of long-term nutritional conditions. It is however worth noting that the majority of Sowetoan children have come into the urban environment with their families in recent years - from rural, invariably homeland environs but also from white farms and 'black spots' threatened with resettlement to Ciskei. The long-term measure - almost half of surveyed children exhibited signs of stunting - is probably a measure of nutritional conditions of the rural home environment from which these families have emigrated.

New Brighton differs from the other communities in that its children generally are well nourished, an impression confirmed by the survey teams. Both present and long-term nutritional conditions are relatively satisfactory, as the results in Tables 10.1 and 10.2 show.

An attempt was also made to establish some measures of child mortality rates in the communities. The mothers or guardians of the children were asked to give the total number of children born to the mother in the last five years and the total number who had died in the same period. The results can only be used as rough estimates of conditions since the survey teams felt this information was unreliable. The results for Tsweletswele were considered completely unsatisfactory but those for the Amatola suggest a mortality rate for children under five of between 77 and 91 per 1,000 live births, for Little Soweto 35 per 1,000 and New Brighton half that of Little Soweto. These are only estimates and reflect the suspicion of the respondents to answering the question. However, what the estimates indicate is an association between nutritional status and mortality rates within communities, with poor nutritional conditions being associated with higher mortality rates.

Socio-Economic Conditions in Surveyed Communities
In this section factors which are associated with nutritional status are considered very briefly. While numerous factors affect nutrition, none is more striking than the availability of family income. However, other factors such as the role of the parents in the household, attitudes of mothers to breastfeeding and access to health care facilities, for example, may also be thought of as important and are considered below.

Figure 10.2 highlights the relationships between nutritional conditions and the access to resources via sufficient incomes. Only New Brighton tops the minimum household subsistence level(HSL), but incomes for both New Brighton and Soweto are far in excess of those in Ciskei. It should be noted that income in kind, not considered in Figure 10.2, may bring in additional resources to the Amatola and Tsweletswele communities.

The surveys revealed that well-organised households in which the father was present and contributing to household income had better nourished children. A major disruption of the functioning of the household occurs through the desertion by either both parents (very uncommon), or the mother (less common) or the father (more common). Migrants to the city may also contribute less and less through time to the rural home. Table 3 depicts, as an example, the role of fathers in Tsweletswele households and the associated nutritional status of children as measured by the presence or absence of oedema, a measure indicating severe nutritional problems in the affected children.

Figure 10.2: Mean Monthly Household Subsistence Level

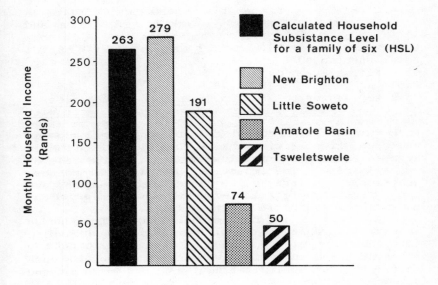

Nutritional Status of Black Communities

Table 10.3 Role of Father in Household, Tsweletswele

Father's status	Child's Nutritional Status			
	Oedemitis No	%	No Oedema No	%	Total No = 100%

Father's status	Oedemitis No	%	No Oedema No	%	Total No = 100%
Commuter	16	33.3	32	66.7	48
Home: Unemployed or informally Employed	10	45.5	12	54.5	22
Deserted/Migrant	28	53.8	24	46.2	52

Fathers who are commuters appear to have fewer children at nutritional risk than those fathers who have deserted the family or migrated away from the 'rural' home. The impact of lack of income is also graphically portrayed by those fathers at home and unemployed or marginally employed and the associated nutritional status of their children.

All communities have mothers who appreciate the value of breast feeding. The children in Amatola for example were kept an average of 18.3 months on the breast and those in New Brighton 7.8 months, the latter shorter period reflecting pressure on mothers to wean the child more quickly to seek work outside the home. It should be noted that New Brighton children are better fed than Amatolan ones which suggests that time spent breast feeding is not a crucial variable. Mothers' nutritional status and other available foods for weaned babies are probably more important.

Clinic attendance for such routine issues as innoculations and the monitoring of weight gains in children is poor in Soweto and Tsweletswele. Only 49 per cent of children in Tsweletswele attended the clinics on a regular basis and 79 per cent from Little Soweto and Tsweletswele which is more an indicator of inadequate facilities than a reticence on the part of consumers to use services. Tsweletswele for instance is serviced by a mobile clinic which visits the settlement once a week. Records of the mobile service indicate that vehicle failure is a problem and the mobile clinic failed to visit Tsweletswele for one full month at one stage.

The survey results indicate that Tsweletswele is clearly the most 'at risk' environment in which to raise children. Amatola children are healthier but the very limited community resource base means that small alterations in environmental conditions can drastically increase the number of children at nutritional risk. Sowetoans live in extremely adverse conditions but the access to employment means that many households are able to raise adequately nourished children. New Brighton children are relatively well nourished and reflect the better socio-economic standing of that community.

NUTRITIONAL INTERVENTION STRATEGIES

It is argued in this section that supplementary feeding, primary health care programmes and nutrition information are crucial ways of tackling the nutritional problems identified. Other important interventions such as food fortification, consumer food price subsidies and agricultural reform are not considered because they are beyond the scope of the chapter. The importance of the political constraints on the development of these communites is another crucial issue which is also unfortunately outside the range of this chapter.
Communities such as Tsweletswele require crisis type interventions. Children with Kwashiorkor or Marasmus, clinically notifiable states, are in grave peril of dying, or at the very least, suffering from severe mental retardation [19,20]. They represent however only the tip of the malnutritional iceberg. While resources must be allocated to their rehabilitation, community and institutional resources need to be increasingly focused on the sub-clinical strata of malnourished children, since it is here that fundamental long-term community problems arise. Many of these children 'survive' the critical first two years of life, but malnourishment during this period invariably has a permanent negative effect on their intellectual and physical development: it precludes them making in later life positive contributions to their group and society in general, and, more importantly, enjoying full and satisfying personal lives.

Supplementary feeding schemes are advocated in the short-term for communities such as Tsweletswele with many malnourished children and insufficient resources to eradicate the problem. The schemes usually aim to tide children over the crucial first two to five years of life (although supplementary feeding of school children is also advocated), while longer term structural changes are anticipated to improve the overall life chances of community members. Bac [21] claims to have had success in intervening at the household level with a supplementary feeding programme in Bophuthatswana, another 'independent' state in South Africa, while clinic and church-based supplementary schemes have sprung up in the Eastern Cape - many in response to the severe drought which is ravaging the area at present. A major problem with these schemes is that they often promote a 'top down' approach to intervention and the schemes end up endorsing community members' (especially mothers of malnourished children) initially low estimation of their own capabilities to help themselves. For supplementary feeding schemes to work, community members must be vitally involved in their operation. One such scheme with a grass roots type approach is the Village Workers Project in Ciskei and Transkei. It is much more than simply a feeding scheme, being an attempt to involve community members as personnel for the administration and administering to the needy in the community. Mothers are taught for example to weigh and to monitor the nutritional status of their own babies, rather than have qualified nursing staff at clinics do these operations for them. The fusing of such grass roots operations to the existing primary health care system could add substantially to efforts to administer feeding programmes successfully.

Work presently being undertaken by the author at the Grahamstown local authority clinics (similar to those found in New Brighton and Soweto) shows that carefully targeted supplementary feeding has a positive impact on weight gains of at risk children. Road to Health Cards, using the Boston norm of weight-for-age provide a suitable monitoring device for such a scheme. The major problem with the feeding scheme is that limited numbers of at risk children are being treated, a common malady of clinic-based feeding schemes [22]. Nursing sisters making house calls in the community report many at risk children. To try and reach these children a type of grassroots programme has been set up using paid personnel and food and money resources extracted from private sponsors. The objective is to offer incentives to mothers and/or the guardians of at risk children to bring their children for feeding. The incentives are in the form of feed for mothers in exchange for performing set tasks in quarters set up at the clinics: for example helping knit woollen blankets or making clothes. Staff hold workshop sessions with these people and try to pinpoint problem areas in raising children; every effort is made to promote better nutrition and hygiene practices among participants. The educative role of the scheme has become important and it is intended to broaden the base of the programme to include a wider spectrum of community mothers and aspirant mothers. A problem which has materialised is that child malnutrition is often the result of mothers falling pregnant by 'mistake' and unwanted children being born. Family planning is therefore a much needed component in any programme aimed at reducing community levels of malnutrition but is a difficult one to integrate into the programme [23].

Whether the feeding scheme takes the scheme products, for example skimmed milk powder, to individual homesteads or is based at clinics, funds are needed to run the programme. A first step - if it is a state institution - is to induce the DOH to put money into such programmes. Experience suggests that it is often slow to do so. Media coverage of health problems is a strategy which can result in action. It is however often the case that the DOH has to compete for funds against other government departments also after the inevitable insufficient pie. It is here that the results of the nutritional surveillance programme are vital in that they provide the Department with the necessary 'scientific facts' to back its call for a greater share of public funds.

The Tsweletswele and Soweto results also point to the gross neglect of these communities by the authorities. Attitudes towards breast feeding for example indicate that mothers of children are only too aware of the need to nurture the young child with care. The often heard call to 'educate' these groups to use scarce resources more advantageously is a nebulous one. Much of their plight is a result of disenfranchisement from the socio-economic and political system, a lack of basic resources and an inadequate health care network, rather than a lack of education.

A measles epidemic swept through Port Elizabeth during 1983. Latest estimates put the number of children who have died at 166 or more than triple the number of deaths reported last year. The majority of these deaths have been in Soweto [24]. The lack of clinic attendance in Soweto, previously mentioned, reflects the inadequate health network in the settlement. The need to broaden out the network of clinics and for preventive and promotive medical activities is essential. Children who are not innoculated against infectious diseases such as measles and are malnourished are at grave risk of early death. What is needed by way of intervention, furthermore, is not piecemeal programmes but an integrated strategy in which primary health care (sanitation, hygiene and family planning) and nutrition are included. For example, measles and other infectious diseases spread in overcrowded, unsanitary communities, while too many children place a burden on scarce household resources resulting in malnourishment which in turn weakens resistance to infection. An integrated strategy is in line with that advocated by Austin et al [25] in which they conceive of such a strategy as a " . . . cluster of health related activities . . . within the context of broader community development efforts". Again, questions of how to fund such activities and who is available to carry out the programmes are raised but not considered here in any detail.

Intervention in New Brighton raises an issue not really important in the other communities. The community has been less troubled by the measles epidemic. Children receive their innoculations, are better fed and so are more capable of withstanding infectious diseases. The nutritional problems in New Brighton are likely to be wide ranging, but one aspect is discussed briefly. Results show that 29 of 205 or 14.4% of children surveyed fall above the 95 percentile of weight-for-age on the NCHS charts and are therefore likely to be overweight. The spectre of overnutrition is a problem ready to emerge within a proportion of the community with satisfactory incomes, flirting with western type foods and diets. The diseases of affluence – predominantly a white trait to date – may strike many of these children in later life [26,27]. In such cases nutrition information is pertinent and should be part of any intervention strategy.

CONCLUSIONS

This chapter has discussed some results of a nutritional surveillance programme in an economically depressed region within South Africa. Results of the surveys reveal a distinction between nutritional conditions of communities studied. Lack of household resources is a key cause of malnutrition. Access to employment opportunities for family members would see a significant reduction in the disease. Since unemployment is likely to remain a problem in communities such as Tsweletswele and Amatola (and Soweto to a lesser extent), carefully targeted outside funds are needed to deal with the problem of malnourishment.

Poverty-stricken communities such as Tsweletswele require crisis intervention in the form of feeding schemes to ameliorate the problems of both Kwashiorkor and undernutrition. Amatola is a rural community forever on the brink of nutrition insufficiency. As with the Tsweletswele and Sowetoan communities, the broadening of the primary health care network of clinics in Amatola can help prevent malnutrition: in times of food scarcity supplementary feeding can be administered from clinics.

Malnutrition is found alongside a range of other community ills. Poor sanitation and overcrowded conditions along with many 'unwanted' children and few household resources are some factors which accentuate the need for integrated programmes of primary health care and nutritional supplementary feeding as part of a preventive health care strategy. Such programmes are crucial in Tsweletswele, Amatola and Soweto. In New Brighton a preventive health care strategy is also important. The need for nutritional education can be given greater prominance; however, since sufficient household resources exist in many cases to fulfil basic nutritional requirements, and wise eating habits need to be encouraged.

The need to have community members committed to strategies to improve conditions within their localities is also vital. While the researcher can be an important advocate of a community's need and at times even a 'broker' between the community and the institutions responsible for their welfare, any intervention attempted without full community consent and participation is unlikely to enjoy the measure of success it deserves.

Finally, a contention of this chapter is that the surveillance programme has been able to differentiate conditions between the communities studied and that it is therefore important to consider the needs of each community separately. In so doing scarce resources allocated or extracted for nutritional intervention can be more wisely used.

REFERENCES

1. Hyman, J. (1979) Baby death rate shocks officials, Daily Dispatch, August 20, pp. 1
2. Gish, O. (1975) Planning the Health Sector: the Tanzanian Experience, Croom Helm, London
3. Newman, J.L. (1980) Dietary behaviour and protein energy malnutrition in Africa South of the Sahara, in M.S. Meade (ed) Conceptual and Methodological Issues in Medical Geography. Studies in Geography No. 15, Department of Geography, University of North Carolina at Chapel Hill
4. Ohuche, R.O. and Otaala, B. (eds) (1981) The African Child and His Environment, Pergamon, Oxford
5. Board, C., Davies, R.J. and Fair, T.J.D. (1970) The structure of the South African space economy: an integrated approach, Regional Studies, Vol. 4, pp. 367-392
6. Fair, T.J.D. (1982) South Africa: Spatial Frameworks for Development, Juta, Cape Town

Nutritional Status of Black Communities

7. Bekker, S., De Wet, C. and Manona, C.W. (1981) A Socio-Economic Survey of the Amatola Basin. Interim Report, Development Studies Working Paper No. 2 , Institute of Social and Economic Research, Rhodes University, Grahamstown
8. Fincham, R.J. (1982) The Nutritional Status of Pre-school Children in the Amatola Basin, Development Studies Working Paper No. 9, Institute of Social and Economic Research, Rhodes University, Grahamstown
9. Mare, G. (1980) African Population Relocation in South Africa, South Africa Institute of Race Relations, Johannesburg
10. Fincham, R.J. (1983) Tsweletswele: Problems and Prospects for Development in a Peri-urban Closer Settlement in Ciskei, Development Studies Working Paper, No. 13, Institute of Social and Economic Research, Rhodes University, Grahamstown
11. Johnston, F.E. (1980) The Causes of Malnutrition, in L.S. Green, and F.E. Johnston (eds) Social and Biological Predictors of Nutritional Status, Physical Growth and Neurological Development, Academic Press, New York
12. Maasdorp, G. (1976) Restructuring the health sector in developing countries, a review article, South Africa Journal of African Affairs, Vol. 1 & 2, pp. 79-86
13. Moosa, A. and Coovadia, H.M. (1981) The problems of malnutrition in South Africa, South African Medical Journal, Vol. 59, No. 25, pp. 888-889
14. Johnston, F.E. (1980) op. cit., pp. 5
15. Hamill, P.V.V. et al (1979) Physical growth, National Center for Health Statistics Percentiles, The American Journal of Clinical Nutrition, Vol. 32, pp. 607-629
16. Hansen, J.D.L. (1979) Assessment of physical growth and development, in R. McDonald, (ed) Growth and Development: A Symposium, Institute of Child Health, University of Cape Town, Cape Town, pp. 1-14

17. Thomas, T. (1980) The effectiveness of alternative methods of managing malnutrition, in Wilson, F. and Westcott, G. (eds) Hunger Work and Health, Economics of Health Care, Vol. 2, Raven Press, Cape Town, pp. 23-46

18. Brown, J.E. and Brown, R.C. (1979) Finding the Causes of Child Malnutrition Task Force and World Hunger, Presbyterian Church, Atlanta, Georgia

19. Cravioto, J. and Robles, B. (1965) Evolution of adaptive and motor behaviour during rehabilitation for Kwashiorkor, American Journal of Orthopedics, Vol. 35, pp. 449-464

20. Hertzig, M.E. et al (1972) Intellectual levels of school children severely malnourished during the first two years of life, Pediatrics, Vol. 49, pp. 814-824

21. Bac, M. (1982) Personal communication with Dr. Bac, Superintendent, Gelukspan Hospital, Bophathatswana

22. McNaughton, J. (1983) Nutrition intervention programmes: pitfalls and potential, Ceres, Vol. 16, pp. 28-33

23. Critical Health, (1983) Contraception, No. 4, May, pp. 63-69

24. From a Report in the Evening Post, 20 May, 1983

25. Austin, J.E. et al (1981) Integrated nutrition and primary health care programmes, in J.E. Austin and M.F. Zeitlin (eds), Nutrition Intervention in Developing Countries, Oelgeschlager, Gunn and Hain, Cambridge, Mass

26. Campbell, G.D. (1973) Statement made in Nutrition and Disease; Hearings before the Select Committee on Nutrition and Human Needs of the United States Senate. U.S. Government Printer, Washington; and

27. Pyle, G.F. (1979) Applied Medical Geography, Wiley, New York

Chapter 11

ETHNICITY AND HEALTH: AN AGENDA FOR
PROGRESSIVE ACTION

Tom Rathwell and David Phillips

INTRODUCTION

Racism is endemic in any society in the sense that
one can always find some cultural group or segment
of that society which finds itself on the receiving
end of some form of abuse, be it overt or covert,
intended or unintended. This book is not about
racism, per se, although racism certainly is
considered to be a factor in determining health care
policies of society as the preceeding papers
testify. This book is about health and minority
groups of which racism is but one factor; albeit
one of crucial importance. The question is really
one of perspective: the argument is not concerned
with racism in health but rather health and
ethnicity. They are very different if related
issues and they are not synonymous.
        Whilst it has been argued that race should not
be regarded as a distinguishing feature between
individuals and/or groups, one is left with a
dilemma of what to replace it with. As this
argument has been extensively rehearsed in chapter
1, it will not be repeated here, except to say
that the use of the terms 'race' and 'ethnicity'
have been used as convenient and familiar
descriptions. It is recognised that application in
such a way does invite criticism but in lieu of any
other suitable and universally acceptable
description it is argued that use of the term 'race'
is appropriate as long as one recognises and accepts
its manifest limitations. Furthermore, it is
contended that discussions on the semantics of
'race' tend to some extent to distort and ultimately
divert attention from the real issue; namely the
provision of a health care network that is sensitive
yet responsive to the particular needs of ethnic
minorities.

The purpose, indeed the crux, of this chapter is the consideration of the many avenues open to both health care policy-makers and providers to realise the global objective of developing "health care services and policies that are sensitive to the specific problems and needs of . . . ethnic minorities" [1]. The manner in which these objectives are achieved will obviously take several forms and operate at different scales from specific national policy initiatives through to local endeavours in response to particular local problems. The range of options is clearly very extensive and the following are presented as possible approaches for consideration.

DEVELOPING POLICY INITIATIVES: A PLANNING FRAMEWORK

Harwood [2] argues that populations who share common origins, identity and standards of behaviour tend to create certain basic concepts and attitudes toward health and illness which, in turn, form that society's bedrock upon which its health care network is developed. Such a philosophy is only valid as long as that society retains its commonality but as soon as it begins to absorb minorities with different cultural backgrounds such assumptions no longer provide the basis for uniform provision. This is of fundamental importance for health care because, according to Harwood, "ethnic differences are . . . of practical concern in treatment situations when patients and providers of care come from different ethnic backgrounds" which often leads to a certain degree of difficulty since "the providers are likely to be unaware of the culturally derived expectations and views of their patients" [3] with the result that providers "may be unable to respond appropriately to the personal needs of patients for information, reassurance and effective treatment" [4].

It is clear from this statement that the development and formulation of health policies for ethnic minorities cannot be undertaken according to the traditional 'western' assumptions for health care and, therefore, an alternative model or, most likely, models of providing such care is/are required. Planning is one such vehicle which has the potential to produce the radical changes in policy necessitated when a society undergoes the transition

An Agenda For Progressive Action

from one which is ethnically and culturally
homogeneous to one that is heterogenous in
composition.
Why this emphasis on health planning as a
crucial determiner of policy? The significance lies
in its ability to evaluate health services "in
relation to the identifiable needs of the community
for different kinds of health care" [5] thereby
establishing planning as an activity which seeks to
distinguish basic health care needs of different
groups in society. Although planning is sometimes
considered to be concerned only with changes in the
patterns of provision, it does have a real value for
both decision-makers and providers because it
focuses not only on what needs doing immediately
but also on that which should be done in the future.
Planning therefore has an important role to perform
because it provides the means through which change
can occur whilst ensuring that such changes accord
with the perceived needs and wishes of the different
communities in society.
The various papers presented in this book have
gone some way to demonstrate that the health
problems of minority groups can be considered under
two separate but not mutually exclusive categories:
illness and ill-health whose manifestations differ
markedly from those of the host population; and the
significant role that culture, religion and language
must play in the determination of suitable and
appropriate policies and programmes. However,
recognising that these are distinct issues affecting
health care programmes and responding positively to
them are two different matters which tend to
reinforce the role of planning. If planning is to be
meaningful and effective in responding to the
particular needs of minority groups, there are at
least six factors which must remain uppermost in the
consideration of policy makers and planners [6].
The first factor concerns cultural differences
and attitudes to health and health care not only
between minority groups and the host population but
also those within minority groups. Such difference
and attitudes are generally acknowledged to be of
importance but in reality they are often little
understood or appreciated by policy-makers, planners
and/or providers [7-9]. A common scenario is one
of mutual bewilderment with the patient unable to
appreciate why he or she is not being responded to
and the doctor unable to understand the meaning of
the symptoms being described.

The second consideration is the seeming lack of trust which many members of minority groups have for doctors and hospitals. This distrust may stem from circumstances which appertained in their country of origin or it could be related to the bureaucratic demands of the health care system which may appear hostile and/or incomprehensible to minority groups. Many members of ethnic groups, for instance, appear to lack the necessary or appropriate documentation with which to obtain health care and often do not understand why such documentation is required. Furthermore, many staff in the health sector do not appreciate the traumatic effect that their demands for the 'right papers' create and they can exacerbate the situation through their often agressive and insensitive behaviour towards minority persons [10]. A frequent consequence of such action is that the hospital ceases to be a place that one seeks for the treatment of illness and instead is associated with the forces of oppression [11].

The third inhibiting feature is the apparent stigma attached by some ethnic or minority groups to particular diseases or illnesses. As in any society there may be certain diseases or illnesses which for some minority groups are taboo and the public admittance of some may result in social ostracism for those concerned. Such consequences may be serious enough for a member of the host or indigenous population but for someone from a minority group the outcome is often doubly damning in the sense that they may feel they are already socially and culturally disadvantaged without having to bear an additional burden related to specific diseases or illnesses. When health care professionals in the majority group are insensitive or unaware of these stigmas or feelings, their treatment or attitudes may be regarded unfavourably by the patient or potential patient. The fourth element concerns the very real barriers imposed on minority groups through differences in life styles, culture and language. Vegetarianism, particularly amongst Asians, is an example of lifestyle that is sometimes relatively little understood and appreciated in Western society. Such attitudes often rebound upon those Asians who use foods not considered to be part of a healthy, well-balanced diet when trying to replicate their more traditional diet. This raises issues of health education in that failure to appreciate the relationships between diet and culture could lead to mis-understanding

over the links to health [12-14]. It can of course
provide problems during periods of hospitalisation
although many institutions now offer sufficiently
flexible vegetarian meal options, if availability is
made clear to patients. Language can also prove to
be a formidable barrier to health care needs
especially in those cases where the husband acts as
interpreter for his wife which can lead to
difficulties with diagnosis as well as the form of
treatment prescribed.
    The fifth constituent deals with the
controversial issue of 'institutionalised
racism' [15], which embodies not only "racist
beliefs but also . . . the power that enables those
who hold such beliefs to engage consciously or
unconsiously in discriminating acts" [16]. McNaught
suggests that racial discrimination against ethnic
minority patients is usually manifested in the
following ways: indifferent and derogatory manner
towards patients by receptionists; clinicians
assuming that ethnic patients exaggerate their
complaints; clinical staff not informing ethnic
patients of the necessity of the procedures;
nursing care that borders on the discriminatory;
and the application of health care models which have
been developed for other groups, to 'explain'
behaviour patterns of ethnic minorities [17]. The
real issue is not whether racial discrimination can
be proved to exist in institutions, rather that most
ethnic minorities believe that it does.
    The sixth, and final, factor relates to the
social and psychological stresses which impact upon
most ethnic minorities as they attempt to adjust or
adapt their previous lifestyles and culture to that
pertaining in their adopted society. Many members
of ethnic minorities are highly vulnerable to
fluctuations in the economic climate since they
often have few marketable skills and inevitably
occupy positions at the lower end of the economic
spectrum. Therefore members of ethnic minorities
not only share many of the social and economic
misfortunes of certain members of the host society,
they also endure specific disadvantages related to
cultural and religious differences, language
problems, traumas associated with immigration, and
the overt and covert presence of racial prejudice
and discrimination. The need for and use of health
care services by ethnic minorities is a function of
their socio-economic and cultural circumstances;
not because they are physically different from the

host   population. As Ballard states "if health care
staff fail to develop a requisite degree of cultural
competence to match their professional skills, they
are bound to get into difficulties with patients who
differ   from   themselves,   and   their therapeutic
effectiveness will necessarily be impaired" [18].
     Participation of health care policy-makers,
planners and providers is therefore a necessity if
any significant changes in the current pattern of
services to ethnic groups are to be forthcoming.
Consequently it is important that all understand and
appreciate how planning functions in order that it
can   be   applied to everyone's mutual benefit.
Health policy-makers, planners and providers are not
omnipotent   -   they   operate   in   an imperfect
environment and their understanding of issues is
only as good as the information available which in
turn influences their perception of and response to
the problems facing them.   The specific task of
health planning is to cultivate the ground so that
the   delivery   of   services   conforms   with the
identified and agreed needs of the consumer; a
function which requires an input and commitment of
all concerned.

A CATALOGUE FOR POSITIVE ACTION

The purpose of this section is to review some of the
initiatives,   either   in   existence   or under
consideration, which could result in a more positive
and progressive pattern of health care for ethnic
minorities.   The range of initiatives described
herein is neither presented as a definitive array of
the sorts of activities nor are options listed in
any order of preference which policy-makers and
providers should undertake, rather they are offered
as examples for discussion when health care policies
for ethnic minorities are in the process of being
formulated.

Communications
Perhaps the most appropriate manner in which to
begin any consideration of policy initiatives would
be with educational programmes directed towards both
health   care   providers   and   ethnic   minority
recipients.   Traditionally, in Britain at least,
such programmes have tended to take the form of
leaflets and other health educational material being

printed in the various languages of ethnic groups. Such approaches, however laudable, have not been without problems, in particular where health educational material originally prepared and produced in English has been directly translated into the appropriate language. Often these attempts at a literal translation create as many or even more problems than they are designed to eliminate because some languages have no direct equivalent of the English term (or terms) such that the message presented can be highly misleading or distorted. There is the additional difficulty that material prepared for the indigenous or host population assumes a degree of familiarity of the health care network, a familiarity that the majority of ethnic groups have not yet achieved. Leaflets which assume this are of little value because they do not provide the sort of information which most ethnic groups need to know.

Communication is not just concerned with providing material in suitable or appropriate languages, it is also about the general demeanour of health staff towards the ethnic patient, and how to ensure full communication with patients who either cannot speak or are largely unfamiliar with the principal language, as these factors can lead to disadvantages and difficulties of access for ethnic groups to health care. Sociologists and cultural geographers have touched on these problems in a range of ways. The problems are not insignificant and although there is no specific package which can be recommended to health care policy-makers and providers, a number of approaches can be commended. Clearly, good interpretation is crucial and therefore it makes sense to employ interpreters well-trained in community languages for which there is considerable demand. For languages of lesser status, a register of staff and/or local people who speak these languages would be of value as would the preparation of leaflets and other material which are well-translated and whose overall purpose would be to help the ethnic patient/consumer to overcome his/her lack of knowledge about and unfamiliarity with the health care network. What, in essence, is being asked of policy-makers and providers is that they must make every effort to see issues from both sides and recognise that the art of communication is a two-way process.

Education and Training
In addition to communication, education and training
is one of the most important areas for making a
dramatic and positive impact upon the welfare of the
ethnic patients. The stress on education and
training is justified, commentators argue, because
it is the only way in which all concerned can become
familiar with and understanding of the special needs
of ethnic minorities [19-21]. The justification for
this focus on education and training is necessary
because it

> involves recognising that because of racial
> discrimination and disadvantage black and
> ethnic minority groups may suffer particular
> inequalities in health, . . . catering for
> differences in culture and language, and
> realising that conscious policy decisions and
> positive health measures may be needed to
> ensure that equality in service provision,
> delivery and employment . . . are
> achieved. [22]

In Britain, attempts to develop training
packages and/or educational material for health
personnel have largely been left to the health
authorities themselves. Consequently any
initiatives have tended to be piecemeal and
localised [23]. One recent development of an
eductional nature is the 'Asians in Britain'
project, a joint venture between the Department of
Health and Social Security, The National Extension
College, and King Edward's Hospital Fund for London.
The main aim of this project has been to develop
and produce, for NHS personnel, training and
educational material relating to Asian people. So
far a book, three booklets and an assortment of
training packs have been produced [24-26]. These
training aids, however valuable, do not often get at
the root of the problem - racial prejudice and
hostility from health service personnel, which may
stem from embarrassment at not understanding the
needs of the patients or misconceptions as to the
value of treating their complaints. Traditional or
standard approaches to the training of health
personnel do not appear to take into account the
problems and the reality associated with any
multi-racial society. Lauridsen's paper (Chapter 7)
provides a useful discussion of the ways in which
Denmark has tackled the challenge of educating all
sides in this question.

In an attempt to counteract 'institutional racism' and to compensate for the lack of attention to racial issues in conventional training programmes the Health Education Council and the National Extension College in Britain launched the Training in Health and Race (THR) project in September 1982, whose remit was to work with NHS personnel in providing training in the different aspects of multi-racial health care for health service workers. One of the major issues arising so far from the THR project has been the production of a checklist Providing Effective Health Care in a Multi-racial Society [27]. The checklist was designed to "provide some practical suggestions on how to improve service provision and promote direct consultation between health authorities and ethnic minority communities" [28]. It accomplishes this objective through an imaginative mix of questions on health care provision, information on the perception of ethnic minorities towards different aspects of health care, and a variety of recommendations and suggestions of good practice. More initiatives of this type should be encouraged because they serve the dual purpose of bringing to the attention of policy-makers, planners and providers the health care implications of a multi-racial society as well as offering specific examples which have been designed to meet the needs of the ethnic community.

Primary Health Care
There is a wealth of literature on ethnic minorities and health which outlines the various health problems encountered by, and manifested in, different ethnic groups [29-31]. Most of the illnesses and diseases apparent amongst ethnic minorities, by and large, lend themselves to the sort of intervention associated with primary health care. In other words, as discussed in chapters 1 and 2, these illnesses and diseases are more a consequence of the environment and the social-economic conditions in which ethnic minorities live, [32] and are not the result of differences in culture or biology [33]. Since the majority of ethnic minorites tend to be "caught in the lowest social classes, with some of the most dangerous and lowest paid jobs, the worst housing and living in some of the worst environmental conditions in the inner cities," [34] primary health care is often an appropriate medium for introducing health practice

263

because of its emphasis on "services that are provided by general practitioners, nurses, health visitors and other staff in the doctors' surgeries, in clinics, in special institutions for the handicapped and impaired and in the patients' home" [35].

Whilst this definition is, to some extent, administratively convenient it does convey a flavour of what primary health care is about, even if the emphasis is essentially on process, content, and location. A detailed discussion of definitions of primary health care is not perhaps the main focus of this chapter, and therefore, whilst acknowledging that the foregoing definition is in many ways imperfect, (excluding, for example, social workers and receptionists) it is nonetheless indicative for what primary health care is generally considered to be in Britain, and it has similar emphasis in a number of other countries.

In short, primary health care might be said to embody not only all institutional activities related to health which are provided at the community level (for example general practitioners, health centres, district nurses), but also those health-related activities carried out by the community (voluntary organisations) and by individuals (friends, neighbours and relatives). To a certain extent the common understanding of primary health care in the United Kingdom sees it as non-hospital care [36]. Perhaps the emphasis should be directed more towards consideration of some of the issues raised by the Alma Ata convention [37], which, important in themselves, become even more so the less homogeneous ethnically a society or community becomes.

The essence of primary health care is that it not only embodies curative methods but also seeks to influence individual behaviour towards health care. The concept also recognises that intervention of a non-health nature, such as an improvement in housing or environmental conditions, may have an equal or greater impact upon a person's or a community's health than that which is purely health oriented. The equation of primary health care with 'holistic' health is also of relevance here. 'Holistic' health implies that not only are the medical components of ill-health treated, so too are its social and cultural attributes. Since it is unrealistic and misleading to expect one person to provide the

comprehensiveness of care such a concept implies, it
is argued that the multi-disciplinary nature of the
primary health care (PHC) team is more suited to the
'holistic' notion of health and health care.

The Primary Health Care Team

The primary health care team is considered to be:

> an interdependent group of general medical
> practitioners and secretaries and/or
> receptionists, health visitors, district nurses
> and midwives who share a common purpose and
> responsibility, each member clearly
> understanding his or her own function and those
> of the other members, so that they all pool
> skills and knowledge to provide an effective
> primary health care service. [38]

The purpose here is not to discuss the
composition or rationale for the PHC team as that
has been done elsewhere [39-41], but to argue that
the responsibilities embodied in the PHC team do
suggest that it has an important and potentially
unique role to play in providing for the health care
needs of ethnic minorities [42].

But perhaps the most important supportive
argument for the PHC team is the interdependence
between the social, cultural, environmental and
physical aspects of health and ill-health and one's
limited understanding of this relationship. The
PHC team by its very ethos seems to be suitably
well-placed to respond in a positive way to the
multivariate facets of health or, at least, has the
potential to do so. This is of particular
relevance in a multi-ethnic society where cultural
differences, especially in relation to one's
perception and understanding of health and illness,
are crucial as they undoubtedly influence any
individual's response to seeking care [43].

Community/consumer Participation

Most commentators support the notion that the path
to better policy formulation and implementation is
one which incorporates the wishes and aspirations of
the community. The logic of such a philosophy is
grounded in the belief that "planning must also be
user-oriented" [44]. That is, the outcome of
policy-making and planning must equate with the
needs and values of the community to which they are
addressed. Despite the accepted rationality of
such a philosophy, the reality of community
participation, particularly in health matters has

been very mixed [45,46]. With respect to ethnic minorities, their participation, as a community in health policy-making and planning has been virtually non-existent [47,48].

It is acknowledged that one of the ways to improving health care for ethnic groups is to encourage their active participation in the decision-making process. Weaver suggests that the best strategy for achieving this is a "partnership of activists and progressive intellectuals. Without the former, the community will be in no position to bargain; without the latter, the government decision-makers will be unreceptive to demands for basic changes" [49]. There is a sense of utopia about such an exhortation because there is a "clear indication of the unwillingness of the system to recognise racial minorities as legitimate consumers" [50]. However, Lauridsen's paper on the experience in Denmark gives some grounds for hope at least in a wealthy country where small minorities may be involved in decision making.

The key to greater consumer or community participation is information. It is crucial because it enables the community or ethnic minorities to argue for better health care from the same base as policy-makers and providers. Information is power and shared information is shared power and it may be more important to arm the client group than just to provide the necessary data to enable the health care professionals to deliver a better service to ethnic minorities. One such forum in Britain for promoting consumer representation in health care is the Community Health Council (CHC) which consists of individuals nominated for their local interest and understanding of health care. McNaught [51] argues that the consumer role of the CHC could be strengthened through internally generated working links with ethnic minority organisations. Others suggest a different form of advocacy, one which gives a greater and more pro-active role to ethnic minorites themselves. Proponents of this type of initiative point to the success of the 'village health worker' in promoting primary health care in developing countries and argue that the concept could be introduced in the developed world as a 'community health worker' drawn from the ethnic minorities, whose responsibilities would be to 'speak' for that minority group, offer advice on the care options available, negotiate if required with health care providers and to help and encourage ethnic minorities in making their particular health needs known to policy-makers and planners [52].

CONCLUSIONS

The initiatives and innovations outlined above will only have a limited impact if developed and implemented in a piecemeal fashion. The absence of clear policy guidelines for health care for ethnic minorities is an important deficiency, and is a situation which must not be permitted to continue for very much longer. The majority of the papers in this volume which described some of the approaches towards providing for or meeting the expressed needs of ethnic minorities document how disparate is the development of health care services for racial minorities.

It is clear from the discussion of the papers and from other informed observers [53], that the time is ripe for a concerted policy intitiative and one which would acknowledge the necessity of incorporating the different values and perspectives of providers, planners and consumers in developing a health care policy for ethnic minorities. This is important because most policy issues, for whatever reason, are generally regarded as single entity issues when in reality they are multifarious and therefore are not conducive to single perspective approaches. Whether the current conservatism of many governments in the western world will encourage positive policies is, of course, debatable.

The role of the planner and policy-maker is crucial here as they are essentially to support those providing patient care. This support is tendered partly through an interpretation of what the issues and problems confronting the providers are perceived to be, and partly by sharing with professionals and consumers the view and concerns of those responsible for the management of the health care organisation. It is the interface between local understanding and knowledge with a frank and open interchange of views which will provide the most appropriate basis for the development and implementation of health programmes relevant to the 'needs' of ethnic communities.

REFERENCES

1. Rathwell, T. (1984) General practice, ethnicity and health services delivery, *Social Science and Medicine*, Vol. 19, No. 2, pp. 123-130
2. Harwood, A. (ed) (1981) *Ethnicity and Medical Care*, Harvard University Press, Cambridge, p. 1
3. Ibid., p. 1
4. Ibid., p. 1
5. Department of Health and Social Security (1972) *Management Arrangements for the Reorganised National Health Service*, HMSO, London
6. Rathwell, T. (1984) op. cit.
7. McNaught, A. (1984) *Race and Health Care in the United Kingdom*, Centre for Health Service Management Studies, Polytechnic of the South Bank, London
8. Torkington, N.P.K. (1983) *The Racial Politics of Health - a Liverpool Profile*, Merseyside Area Profile Group, Department of Sociology, University of Liverpool, Liverpool
9. Weaver, J.L. (1976) *National Health Policy and the Underserved*, C.C. Mosby Co., St. Louis
10. Torkington, N. (1983) op. cit.
11. Rathwell, T. (1984) op. cit.
12. Henley, A. (1979) *Asians: Patients in Hospital and at Home*, DHSS/King Edward's Hospital Fund for London, London
13. Henley, A. (1982) *Caring for Muslims and their Families*, DHSS/King Edward's Hospital Fund for London, London
14. Henley, A. (1983) *Caring for Sikhs and their Families*, DHSS/King Edward's Hospital Fund for London, London
15. Torkington, N. (1983) op. cit.
16. Ibid.
17. McNaught, A. (1984) op. cit.
18. Ballard, R. (1983) *The Implications of Cultural Diversity for Medical Practice; An Anthropological Perspective*, Unpublished paper
19. McNaught, A. (1984) op. cit.
20. Greater London Council (undated) *The National Health Service and Ethnic Minorities*, Report 20.1082, Greater London Council, London

21. Health   Education   Council/National   Extension
        College for Training in Health and Race
        (1984) Providing Effective Health Care in
        a Multiracial Society, Training in Health
        and Race, London
22. Ibid., pp. 3
23. McNaught, A. (1984) op. cit.
24. Henley, A. (1979) op. cit.
25. Henley, A. (1983) op. cit.
26. Henley. A. (1984) Caring for Hindus and their
        Families, DHSS/NEC/King's Fund, London
27. HEC/NECTHR (1984) op. cit.
28. Ibid., pp. ii
29. Johnson, M.R.D. (1983) Race and Health: a
        Selected Bibliography, SSRC Research Unit
        on Ethnic Relations, University of Aston,
        Birmingham
30. Donovan, J.L. (1984) Ethnicity and health:
        a research   review,   Social Science and
        Medicine, Vol. 19, pp. 663-670
31. Johnson, M.R.D.   (1984) Ethnic minorities
        and   health, Journal Royal College of
        Physicians, London, Vol. 18, No.4, pp.
        228-230
32. Brent Community   Health   Council   (1981)
        Black People and the Health Service, Brent
        CHC, London
33. Johnson, M. (1984) op. cit.
34. Donovan (1984), op. cit. pp. 669
35. Hicks, D. (1976) Primary Health Care, HMSO,
        London
36. Metcalfe, D. (1982) Flexible doctoring, The
        Health Services, May, pp. 20
37. World Health Organisation (1978) Primary Health
        Care,   Report   of   the   International
        Conference on Primary Health Care, Alma
        Ata, USSR, September, WHO, Geneva
38. Harding Report (1981) The Primary Health Care
        Team, Report of a Joint Working Group of
        the Standing Medical Advisory Committee
        and the Standing Nursing and Midwifery
        Advisory Committee, London
39. Rathwell, T. (1984) op. cit.
40. Harding (1981) op. cit.
41. Phillips, D.R. (1981) Contemporary Issues in
        the Geography of Health Care, Geo Books,
        Norwich
42. Rathwell, T. (1984) op. cit.
43. Runnymede Trust and Radical Statistics Race
        Group (1980) Britain's Black Population,
        Heinemann, London

44. Gans, H.J. (1972) *Plans and People*, Penguin, Harmondsworth, pp. xi
45. Lee, K. and Mills, A (1982) *Policy-making and Planning in the Health Sector*, Croom-Helm, London
46. Checkoway, B. (ed) (1981) *Citizens and Health Care. Participation and Planning for Social Change*, Pergamon, New York
47. McNaught, A. (1984) op. cit.
48. Torkington, N. (1983) op. cit.
49. Weaver, J. (1976) op. cit., pp. 148
50. Torkington, N.P.K. (1983) op. cit. pp. 72
51. McNaught, A. (1984) op. cit.
52. Winkler, F. (1983) Advocacy in health: racial minorities and maternity services, *Radical Community Medicine*, No.16, Winter, pp. 51-54
53. Harwood, A. (1981) op. cit.

INDEX

Aboriginies, Australian
    25
accidents 50
addiction 51, 58
aetiology 82
Afghanistan 41
air pollution 50
Airedale   Health
District 89, 91, 96
alcoholism 50, 51
allopathic 12
Alma Ata 265
alternative
    practitioner   211
American   Medical
    Association 61, 64,
    65,
anaemia   25,   190,
    iron deficiency 96
    sickle   cell 6, 26
    135,   194
    thalassaemia   135
antenatal   care   113
anthropologist 9, 23,
    26
ante-immigration
    campaign 41
anti-racist   movement,
    history 33-41
Arneil, G. and Crosbie,
    J. 120
Asian   Mother and Baby
    Campaign 102
artherosclerosis   45,
    58
Australia 58, 139
Ayurvedic   medicine
    12

Ayurvedic   practitioner
    210
Bac, M. 250
Baker, M. 210,
Ballard, R. 262,
Beri beri 242,
biological determinism 22
Binding,   and   Hoche
    65,
Birmingham 195, 196
    Inner   City
    Partnership 195
Black Report 118
blood   pressure 25, 47,
    52, 126
Blue Cross 222
Boal, F.W. 147
body mass index 25
Bolivia 58
Bophuthatswana 250
Boyd, W.C. 31
Bradford 93, 112, 211
Bradford Health District
    13, 90-98 passim
Bradford   Metropolitan
    District   89,   92
breast cancer 48
Brent   Community   Health
    Council 122
Brown,   J.E. and Brown,
    R.C. 244
bronchitis 190
Boston   (Harvard)
    anthropometric
    measurements 240
Buffon 24, 27, 40
Bujra, J. 2

Canada 58,
cancer 26, 43, 52, 58
    breast 48
    cervix 85
    leukaemia 48
    lung 48, 50
    prostatic 48
capitalism 29,   51,
    103
    European 32
carcinogens, pulminary
    48
cardiovascular disease
    46
Carlyle, T. 2
carotene intake   48,
    50
cause-specific analysis
    52
Chicago 146, 147, 157,
    168
Chicago   Regional
    Hospital Study 10
cirrhosis 50
civil   rights
    legislation 62
clinical   psychiatry
    149
Cochrane, R. 143
Collins, E. and Klein,
    R.   207
Commonwealth Immigrants
    Act 122
communications 262-3
Community   Health
    Councils (CHC) 268
community care 7, 8
community/
    participation 267-9
community   relations
councils 101
consumer participation
    267-9
Coon, C.S. 26, 31
coronary heart disease
    43, 45, 51, 88, 94-
    6
cost-benefit   analysis
    63
Coventry 196, 198

culture
    common   themes
    111-3
    difference of 106-8
cultural pluralism   104-
    6
cystic fibrosis 135

Denmark
    Association of Health
    Professionals   181
    Association of County
    Councils 183
    Council   of   Migrants
    185, 187
    ethnic groups 178-9
    health care and ethnic
    minorities 177-93
    health policy 183-4
    health system 180-3
    general   migration
    policy 186-8
    Ministry of Education
    180
    Ministry   of   the
    Interior   180,   184,
    187
    national   health
    insurance 181
    National   Council   of
    Prevention 180
    National Institute for
    Social Research 188
    political   and
    administrative   system
    179-80
    Social Science Research
    Council 189
    State   University
    Hospital 180
dental caries 85
Department of Health and
    Social Security 102
    120, 264
    Asian Mother and Baby
    Campaign   102
    Rickets Campaign 102
Diabetes 51, 126
diarrheal disease   59,
    61

Index

differential mortality,
mechanisms   51-2
dietary   difficiences
120
dietary factors   47
Diphtheria   93
Dobzhansky,   T.   25,
26
Durkheim, E.   2

Eastern   Cape,   South
Africa
socio-economic
conditions   246-9
ecological   analysis
146-8
ecological   psychiatry
146,   149
ecological   studies,
psychiatric   146
education   219
elderly   8, 41
end-stage renal disease
51
environment   81
environmental   hazards,
lead   96-7
epidemiological
research,
psychiatric   146
epidemiology
concepts of   82-7
definition of   82
erythrocyte
protoporphyrin   96
ethnic   groups, health
differences   4, 81
ethnic minorities
health care   11
special   care groups
11
ethnic   relations
studies   103-8
ethnicity   and
schizophrenia,
Nottingham   148-68
euthanasia   63
Evans, R.W.   65

experimentation
random control
designs   83

facism   67
Faris, R. and Dunham, H.
146, 147, 157, 168
fluoridation   83
folk medicine   211

gastro-intestinal
infections   92-3
dysentry 93
paratyphoid 92
shigella dysenteria
92
shigella flexneria   92
shigella sonnei   92
typhoid   89, 92
gender   41
general practitioners (GP)
196-208
genotype   28
geography   139
geographical inequalities
211
Glass, B.   27
Gobineau, A. De   1

haemoglobin   25, 96
haemophilia   135
hakims   12, 135, 211
Haldanes dilemma   28
Hansen, J.D.L.   243
Hare, E.H.   157
Hart, J.T.   87
Harvard (Boston)
anthropometric
measurements   240
Harwood, A.   258
health
determinants of   84
economists   9
status   4, 52
health and illness   125-7
health-care   132-4
Health Education Council
265
health planning
definition   259

Index

heart disease 43
Hepatitis 'B' virus
    102
herbalist 211
Herbert, R.T. and
    Thomas, C.J. 11
high blood pressure
    126
holistic medicine
    210
homicide 50,51
human biology 81
Husband, C. 3
hypertension 25, 43-56
    passim, 126
Hypertension Detection
    and Follow-up
    Program 46

Immigration Act 122
infant mortality 53
infectious diseases
    childhood 93-4
    diphtheria 93
    measles 93, 210,
    252
    rubella 93
    tuberculosis 6, 51,
    58, 82-110 passim,
    119, 123, 135
    typhoid 89, 92
    whooping cough 93
    venereal 51, 19
Inner City Partnership,
    Birmingham 195
international
    anthropometric
    norms 243
International
    Classification
    of Diseases (ICD)
    153-6 passim
International Committee
    Against Racism 36
inverse care law 87
iron deficiency anaemia
    96
Ischaemic heart disease
    85, 95

Italy
    gross national
    product 59

Japan,
    cast system 58
Johnson, M.R.D. 6
Johnston, F.E. 243
Jones, P.N. 152
Joseph, A.E. and Phillips,
    D.R. 11

King Edward's Hospital
    Fund for London 264
Knox, P.L. 11
Kwashiorkor 242, 243, 249
    253

Lebanon 41
Leeds University,
    Department of Community
    Medicine 87
Leibel, R. 63
Leicester 113
leukaemia 48
Levy, L. and Rowitz, L.
    157, 168
Lewontin, R.C. 27
life expectancy 56
life-style 81, 88, 120
Lilianfeld, D.E. 82
lipoproteins 43
London 211
low birthweights 119
lung cancer 48, 50

Marasmus 242, 249
Marx, K. 23, 31
Masai 25
malnutrition 240, 241,
    250
    measurement of 242-3
McNaught, A. 6, 16, 261,
    268
McNeely, R.L. and Cohen,
    J.L. 8
measles 93, 210, 252
Medicaid 62, 64, 215,
    222
Medicare 215

274

Index

medical
  geography 157
  geographers 7
  ideology 108-11
  model 7
  sociologists 9
medical geography
  health and health
  care 10-3
mental disorders
  ethnic status 140
  scientific
  investigation 139
  senile psychoses
  145
  schizophrenia
mentally handicapped
  8
mental health 119
mental illness 81
  ethnic status 139
mentally ill 8
Michigan 14, 215-8,
  222-9 passim, 232-3
Michigan Department of
  Public Health 219
Michigan Health Data
  Corporation 216
migrant workers,
  Denmark 178-9
Montague, A. 31
morbidity 219
mortality 43,46, 58
  structure of 52
  infant 53, 97-8
  perinatal and infant
  97-8
Myrdal, G. 33, 34

National Extension
  College 264
National Health Service
  5, 9, 85, 194
National Center for
  Health Services
  Research 217
National Center for
  Health Statistics
  Percentiles (NCHS)
  243, 252
Nationality Act 122

neo-colonial countries
  58
neoplastic diseases
  48
Newsholme, A. 28
New Zealand 58
Non-hierarchical cluster
  analysis 160
Nordic Council of
  Ministers 189
Nottingham 15, 140-68
  passim
  ecological structure
  155-68
  ethnicity and
  schizophrenia 148-68
Nottingham Psychiatric
  Case Register (NPCR)
  139, 148-68 passim
nutritional assessment
  243-6
nutritional intervention
strategies 249-53
Nutritional Surveillance
  Programme 238, 241,
  251

obesity 25, 52
osteomalacia 194

paranoia 121, 152
paratyphoid 92
pelagra 242
perinatal and infant
  mortality 97-8
phenotype 28
Phillips, D.R 206
phlogiston 29
pica 96
population genetics 48
poverty 219-20
  culture of 34
Preston, S.H. 59
preventive medicine 208-
  10
primary health care 15,
  252-3, 265-7
primary health care team
  267
principal components
  analysis 160

275

Index

Progressive Labour
    Party   35
prostatic cancer   48
protein   energy
    malnutrition   (PEM)
    242
psychiatric   disorders
    51
psychiatric ecological
    studies 146
psychiatric
    epidemiology   144-6
    morbidity 143
    relevant   problems
    142-4
    services 154
psychosomatic 83
public health 22
pulmonary tuberculosis
    85, 88

quality of care   195

race
    concept of   23-31
    class question 31-
    41
    definition 1
    public health   28-
    31
    social concept 29
    social construct 2
race and biology
    historical view 23-
    8
race relations
    policies 16
    studies 103-8
racial determinism 2
racial discrimination,
    manifestations
    261
racial inequality
    health 22
racism 129-32
    class weapon 36
    institutional 104
    origins of 31-3
Rathwell, T. 11
Reich, M., 36, 53, 56

research
    agenda for 114-5
    cultural   pluralistic
    114
    cultural   studies
    115
    policy-oriented 114
    mental heath 120
    role of   113-4
respiratory disease 190
rickets   6,   119, 121,
    135, 190. 194
Rickets Campaign 102
Rhodes University 238
Rockefeller   Foundation
    61
Rogers, D.E.   64
rubella 93

Schizophrenia   15,   119,
    121,   140, 142, 145,
    152-68 passim
    incidence   of,
    Nottingham 152-6
senile psychoses 145
serum allumin levels 45,
    46
serum cholesterol levels
    45, 46
shigella dysenteriae 92
shigella flexneri 92
shigella sonnei 92
sickle-cell   anaemia   6,
    26, 119, 135
slavery, origins of racism
    31-3
smallpox 210
social biology 9
social engineering 23
social environment 47
social injustice 10
social justice 10, 11
Society for the Study of
    Social Biology 9
sociological   inequalities
    211
sociologists 9
    medical   9

Index

South Africa
    Eastern Cape 15,
    238, 241-2
    Institute of Social
    and Economic
    Research 238
    Rhodes University,
    238
still-births 98
Stone, J. 2
suicide 43
super-exploitation
    36, 51, 53
surma 96

Third World 12
Thomas, T. 243
Tosteson, D. 64
Training in Health and
    Race 265
traditional healers
    12, 135
traditional medicine
12
tuberculosis 6, 51
    58, 82-110 passim,
    119, 123, 135
typhoid 89, 92

Unani medicine 12
Unani practitioners
    210
ultra-violet radiation
    120
unemployment 51, 110,
    112, 219
United Kingdom
    Airedale Health
    District 89, 91,
    96
    Bradford Health
    District 13, 90-8
    passim
    Bradford
    Metropolitan
    District 89, 92
    Centre for Research
    on Ethnic Relations
    15,

    see Department of
    Health and Social
    Security
    Health Education
    Council 265
    King Edward's Hospital
    Fund for London 264
    Leeds University,
    Department of Community
    Medicine 86
    National Extension
    College 264, 265
    see National Health
    Service
    Nottingham 15, 140-68
    passim
    Nottingham Psychiatric
    Case Register 139,
    148-68
    Training in Health and
    Race 265
    Warwick University 15,
    West Midlands 15, 195
    West Yorkshire 94
United States of America
    American Medical
    Association 61, 64,
    65
    Blue Cross 222
    Chicago Regional
    Hospital Study 10
    Communist Party 33, 35
    gross national product
    59
    Medicaid 62, 64, 215,
    222
    Medicare 215
    Michigan 14, 215-8,
    222-9 passim, 232-3
    Michigan Department of
    Public Health 219
    Michigan Health Data
    Corporation 216
    race and hospital use
    215-6
    racism and health care
    services 61-7
    Rockefeller Foundation
    61

277

Index

urban social ecology
157

vaids 12, 211
venereal disease 51,
119
victim-blaming 103
violence 50, 52, 58
culture of 50
vitamin D deficiency
120

Watt, E.S 24
Webb, P. 122
Weightman, G. 211
West Midlands 15,
195
primary health care
15
West Yorkshire 94
western medicine
history and ideology
108-11
mechanistic 108-9
scientific 108-9
whooping cough 93
Wilson, E.O. 31, 40
Wing, J.K. 154
work and health 127-9
World Health
Organization 86,
88,
Wolverhampton 196,
203

Zubaida, S. 1